"*The Anxiety Skills Workbook*, by world-leading expert on anxiety Stefan Hofmann, is an excellent, up-to-date guide for those suffering from anxiety. Following the clear, powerful, and concise techniques outlined in each chapter, the reader will have all the tools needed to conquer anxiety. Step by step, you will learn how to acquire skills in relaxation, mindfulness, challenging negative thoughts, coping with worry, and confronting avoidance. Each chapter provides easy-to-use exercises that can help you reverse your anxiety. This book will make a difference in your life!"

—**Robert L. Leahy, PhD**, director of the American Institute for Cognitive Therapy, and author of *The Jealousy Cure*

"Millions of people in North America and around the world spend billions of dollars each year in vain attempts to suppress and escape the ravages of severe anxiety. In this brief, easy-to-read workbook, one of the foremost authorities on anxiety in the world, Stefan Hofmann, lays out several relatively simple, straightforward, and proven strategies based on the latest cutting-edge research to face life's daily challenges with confidence rather than fear. By individually tailoring these strategies to their own situation, everyone suffering from anxiety should benefit."

—**David H. Barlow, PhD, ABPP**, professor of psychology and psychiatry emeritus, and founder of the Center for Anxiety and Related Disorders at Boston University

"This workbook could be a game changer for those struggling with anxiety. It is packed full of the latest evidence-based knowledge and treatment strategies that target key symptoms of anxiety. Written by Stefan Hofmann, a world-renowned researcher and clinician in the treatment of anxiety disorders, *The Anxiety Skills Workbook* presents modular, step-by-step instruction on how to deal with the root causes of persistent anxiety. Readers will find the case examples, uncomplicated worksheets, and straightforward explanations a refreshing departure from a crowded field of self-help books on anxiety."

—**David A. Clark, PhD**, professor emeritus in the department of psychology at the University of New Brunswick in Canada, and author of *The Anxious Thoughts Workbook*

"Tens of millions of people have benefitted from cognitive and behavioral therapies to develop a new relationship with anxiety. Stefan Hofmann is a world-leading scientist and practitioner, and presents here an easy-to-use anxiety skills workbook that is firmly grounded in the latest research. The evidence is clear: it's not what happens to us, but rethinking the ongoing stresses and events that happen in life, as well as our beliefs about emotions, worry, and replacing past memories with experiences of accomplishment in tricky situations that helps us to grow. Anyone wanting to alleviate their anxiety should read this book."

—**Nikolaos Kazantzis, PhD**, associate professor at Monash University in Australia,
coauthor of *The Therapeutic Relationship in Cognitive Behavioral Therapy*,
and coeditor of *Using Homework Assignments in Cognitive Behavior Therapy*

"Many self-help books tend to overwhelm readers with endless lists of worksheets to be completed, and suggestions for too many 'homework exercises.' This book is refreshingly different. It helps readers to quickly zero in on the most important issues common to all anxiety problems. Each chapter teaches the reader just a few exercises that were carefully selected based on what the latest scientific research has shown repeatedly to be effective in the treatment of anxiety. Rather than feeling like victims of anxiety, these exercises will empower readers to move with anxiety rather than struggling against it, thus making them feel less like victims of anxiety and more in charge of their lives. If you're looking for a bare-bones workbook to help you deal with anxiety more effectively, this workbook will be perfect for you."

—**Georg H. Eifert, PhD**, professor emeritus of psychology at Chapman University,
and coauthor of *The Mindfulness and Acceptance Workbook for Anxiety*

"Stefan Hofmann is an expert in the areas of anxiety, fear, and worry, and his outstanding book will teach you how to help yourself with cognitive behavioral as well as mindfulness treatment strategies. This book is filled with clear and practical advice that will guide your journey toward a better life."

—**Sabine Wilhelm, PhD**, professor at Harvard Medical School,
and chief of psychology at Massachusetts General Hospital

"This book combines a range of effective strategies that have been studied for decades with newer approaches for understanding and treating anxiety and related problems. It's clearly written, well organized, and filled with helpful tips and tools to stop anxiety in its tracks. The best way to overcome anxiety is to change the thoughts and behaviors that keep it alive. This book will show you how to do exactly that. I recommend it highly!"

—**Martin M. Antony, PhD, ABPP**, professor in the department of psychology at Ryerson University in Canada, and coauthor of *The Shyness and Social Anxiety Workbook*

"If you are anxious, you know your problem from the inside out—so why use a one-size-fits-all approach if you can instead learn to do what fits your needs? Written by one of the world's leading experts on cognitive behavioral approaches to emotion, this workbook takes some of the most effective skills for addressing anxiety and breaks them down into bite-sized modules that you can learn and use either as an overall package or as stand-alone strategies. Research suggests that these modules—these micro-skills—are highly effective and worth your effort to learn. Highly recommended."

—**Steven C. Hayes, PhD**, Foundation Professor in the department of psychology at the University of Nevada, Reno

The

Anxiety Skills
Workbook

Simple CBT and Mindfulness Strategies for Overcoming Anxiety, Fear, and Worry

STEFAN G. HOFMANN, PhD

New Harbinger Publications, Inc.

Publisher's Note

Printed in the United States of America

Distributed in Canada by Raincoast Books

Copyright © 2020 by Stefan G. Hofmann
        New Harbinger Publications, Inc.
        5674 Shattuck Avenue
        Oakland, CA 94609
        www.newharbinger.com

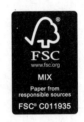 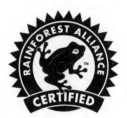

Cover design by Sara Christian

Acquired by Elizabeth Hollis Hansen

Edited by Karen Levy

Library of Congress Cataloging-in-Publication Data

Names: Hofmann, Stefan G., author.
Title: The anxiety skills workbook : simple CBT and mindfulness strategies for overcoming anxiety, fear, and
    worry / Stefan G. Hofmann, PHD ; foreword by Judith S. Beck, PHD.
Description: Oakland, CA : New Harbinger Publications, [2020] | Includes bibliographical references.
Identifiers: LCCN 2019055161 (print) | LCCN 2019055162 (ebook) | ISBN 9781684034529 (paperback) |
    ISBN 9781684034536 (pdf) | ISBN 9781684034543 (epub)
Subjects: LCSH: Anxiety disorders--Treatment. | Cognitive therapy.
Classification: LCC RC531 .H64 2020 (print) | LCC RC531 (ebook) | DDC 616.85/2206--dc23
LC record available at https://lccn.loc.gov/2019055161
LC ebook record available at https://lccn.loc.gov/2019055162

Printed in the United States of America

22   21   20

10   9   8   7   6   5   4   3   2   1   First Printing

To our courageous clients, who have taught us so much.

Contents

Foreword

Anxiety and worries are common emotional problems. For some people, these problems are so severe that they lead to a great degree of stress and suffering. We know a great deal about the nature of these problems, and there are many books on anxiety and worry. But simply knowing the facts about anxiety and worry is unlikely to change much. Similarly, passive advice about common treatment strategies that should work for most, as happens with so many self-help books, will not lead to success. Rather, success comes from actively working to identify and change the unhelpful patterns *of the unique individual*. This point is a distinctive feature of this book, unshared by others. It consists of treatment *modules* that focus on different aspects of anxiety. Not all modules will be equally beneficial for everyone. Such a modular approach toward overcoming anxiety recognizes the unique problems any given client is facing. Matching the right modules to these problems is the most powerful way to target and overcome anxiety.

The workbook starts by encouraging readers to think critically about their reasons for wanting to change and to develop concrete goals about what that change will look like. This is a critical step that is too often neglected, as having something tangible to strive for makes doing the work required for reducing one's anxiety feel much more manageable.

The general framework of the book is based on the cognitive behavioral model of anxiety. This model is supported by decades of research on tens of thousands of anxious patients. It teaches us how thoughts, behaviors, and physical sensations interact to create a vicious cycle of anxiety that can make us feel trapped. This model serves as the framework for the skills taught throughout the rest of the book, with each subsequent module covering strategies for targeting one of these three anxiety components.

The "Mindful Relaxation" module teaches us about how to achieve physical and mental relaxation. Often, anxiety involves physical tension and a busy mind; these require specific techniques to promote relaxation. The book does an excellent job of teaching readers progressive muscle relaxation, a strategy that promotes deep relaxation throughout different body parts, as well as mindfulness, which can help people be more focused on the present moment.

The "Rethinking Thoughts" module focuses on biased thinking patterns in maintaining anxiety. More importantly, readers will learn specific strategies for responding to dysfunctional thoughts and generating more realistic and helpful thinking patterns. Cognitive restructuring is a fundamental strategy in the cognitive behavioral tradition, and there is a wealth of scientific evidence supporting its effectiveness. The book provides clear instructions and useful examples to assist readers in teaching themselves these foundational strategies for overcoming problematic anxiety.

The "Worries About Worries" module teaches readers a number of strategies that can help them get more distance from anxious thoughts. These strategies come from recent research and work in the clinic that shows that it's not just thoughts that drive anxiety, but also the way we think about our thoughts. Exercises are designed to show that such thoughts about thoughts, or metacognitions, tend to be inaccurate. The module teaches alternative ways of responding to anxious thoughts that allow more freedom to focus on what's important to us.

The "Facing Feared Scenarios and Images" module presents the groundwork on how to overcome and face fearful thoughts and scenarios. Often, anxiety encourages people to avoid what they fear most, whether it's an object, a place, or an image. Readers will learn how to conquer their scariest thoughts by learning how to use mental imagery to gradually expose themselves to their worst-case scenarios.

The focus on intolerance of uncertainty in the "Changing Behaviors" module is critical, as uncertainty is an unavoidable part of daily life and only appears to be increasing in our ever-evolving busy world. We are ultimately faced with the choice of continuing to try to fruitlessly gain more certainty or to do the challenging work of bolstering tolerance of uncertainty through the behavioral change exercises presented in this module. The book does an excellent job of guiding the reader through designing their own behavioral change activities and learning how to monitor the process and tweak them as needed.

Another excellent part of this workbook is the way the exercises build off each other and can be individualized based on the reader's situation. In the final module, "Progress on Goals and Relapse Prevention," readers get the opportunity to review everything they have learned and create a plan to maintain and build upon their gains.

—Judith S. Beck, PhD
Director, Beck Institute

Contributing Authors

The following individuals served as coauthors of this workbook and therapists of the treatment:

Amanda Baker, PhD, is a clinical psychologist at the Center for Anxiety and Traumatic Stress Disorders at Massachusetts General Hospital (MGH) and assistant professor at Harvard Medical School (HMS). Dr. Baker received her PhD from Boston University and completed her predoctoral internship and postdoctoral training at MGH/HMS. Her clinical and research interests involve mediators and moderators of cognitive behavioral treatments for anxiety. In 2018 she completed a KL2/CMeRIT Harvard Catalyst/The Harvard Clinical and Translational Science Center/National Institutes of Health grant and in 2019 she was awarded a NARSAD award. She has expertise in evidence-based therapies for anxiety, mood, obsessive-compulsive spectrum, and traumatic stress disorders.

Joseph K. Carpenter, MA, is a doctoral candidate in clinical psychology at Boston University, and at the time of publication is completing his internship at the VA Boston, where he provides clinical services for veterans with trauma-related difficulties. He has expertise in the delivery of cognitive behavioral therapy for anxiety and related disorders, and conducts research aimed at improving treatments for such conditions. His research focuses on translating insights from basic research on fear, learning, and memory into novel therapeutic approaches for treating anxiety.

Joshua E. Curtiss, MA, is a doctoral researcher at Boston University, completing a doctoral internship at Harvard Medical School–Massachusetts General Hospital (MGH/HMS). Previously, he conducted psychology research at Yale University as a statistician. His interests include the use of innovative statistical modeling to address issues pertaining to the treatment and nosology of emotional disorders. He is also the author of another popular book on anxiety disorders published by New Harbinger (*Don't Let Anxiety Run Your Life*).

Elizabeth M. Goetter, PhD, is a clinical psychologist at the Center for Anxiety and Traumatic Stress Disorders at Massachusetts General Hospital (MGH) and assistant professor at Harvard Medical School (HMS). She also serves as codirector of the Red Sox Foundation and MGH Home Base Program's Outpatient Clinic. Dr. Goetter received her PhD from Drexel University.

She completed her predoctoral internship at the University of California, San Diego/VA San Diego Healthcare System and received her postdoctoral training at MGH/HMS. Her clinical specialty is in the evidence-based treatment of anxiety and trauma and stressor-related disorders. She has worked as an independent evaluator and study therapist on multiple NIH-, NIMH-, and DOD-funded studies.

Prologue

Are you a worrier? Are you more anxious than most people? Is your anxiety controlling your life? Are you missing out on life because of your anxiety and worries? You are not alone. Anxiety and anxiety disorders are some of the most common psychological problems. They cause a great degree of suffering and keep people from reaching their goals and living a fulfilled, meaningful, and happy life. If anxiety holds you back and keeps you trapped, this book will point you to the way out of your misery. If you follow our advice, we firmly believe you'll successfully be able to transform your life by transforming your anxious mind.

Why are we so confident that we can help you? Because we know it works! We are clinical scientists and experts in mood and anxiety disorders, working for decades as front-line clinicians with the most severe forms of stress, mood, and anxiety disorders. The techniques outlined in this book comprise the concrete strategies that any competent clinician needs to know to treat anxiety problems. They've been developed during decades of rigorous clinical research and countless clinical trials and studies, resulting in the concrete evidence-based practices outlined in this book. It took many great thinkers and clinicians to develop these strategies—too many to name them here in detail. This book translates these insights and techniques into a relatively easy how-to guide to reclaim your life.

This is probably not the first book on anxiety you've held in your hands. We know that the self-help literature for anxiety problems can feel overwhelming and confusing, and unfortunately many of these books are ill informed. You might have also tried getting help for your problems from a counselor or a psychiatrist. Similarly, many counselors you've encountered may not have been overly helpful because they haven't been trained in the best techniques for anxiety. There are also many reasons why medication might not be a good idea for you. We can recommend the techniques in this book for everyone because the research has shown how widely they help. If you haven't tried them yet, we strongly urge you to give it a shot. You don't have anything to lose, and we're confident they will help.

At the same time, no two people are alike. Each of us has a unique history. Our bodies and minds respond in unique ways to the same situation. We differ in our weaknesses and our strengths. Therefore, there is no *single* approach that will target *all* anxiety problems for *all* people. Rather, there are some strategies that work very well for some people and other strategies that work well for others. This is why the one-size-fits-all method of most self-help books is usually met with disappointment. Instead, we need to find the *right* strategy that fits to solve the problem for *you*.

For this reason, we've devised treatment modules to deal with your anxiety and worry. Each module targets a different aspect of your problem. These modules are related, but they can also be used as stand-alone strategies. Nobody knows your problem better than you do. You are your own best expert, so you'll be in the best position to decide what works for you. We advise you to work through the entire book and all modules in a step-by-step fashion first, but to then come back to the modules that have worked the best for you. Once you've figured out which strategies work the best, hold on to them and keep practicing. You'll see dramatic results in only a few weeks. Go ahead. Try it out. Transform your life. Transform your anxious mind.

How to Use This Workbook

Congratulations! By opening up this workbook, you've taken the first step toward doing something about your anxiety. Although this might seem trivial, it's no small feat. Anxiety affects over a quarter of the population, yet many people go for years without addressing it, and some never do anything about it at all. There are a number of understandable and relatable reasons for this. Many people are afraid to acknowledge their anxiety or feel self-conscious admitting it to other people. Others may think anxiety is something they have to live with, and that there isn't anything that can be done. Still others have no idea where to look for help or find the process to be too overwhelming. And, sometimes, people simply don't realize the extent to which anxiety makes their life more difficult. You might have had a number of these thoughts yourself. The fact that you're reading this right now, however, means that you're on your way to dealing with your anxiety differently, and that's a good reason to feel hopeful!

Another reason for you to feel hopeful is that the authors of this book know, from working with hundreds of people suffering from anxiety, that anxiety can be effectively treated. A major goal of this workbook is to show you that intense anxiety and worry isn't something you simply have to deal with. Rather, there are a number of tools and strategies that you can learn to significantly reduce the impact it has on your life. These changes might not happen overnight, but with consistent practice, the tools you'll learn can change the relationship you have with anxiety. Rather than anxiety controlling you, you can control how you respond to anxiety, and move closer toward living the life that you want.

Is This Book Right for You?

Anxiety is a universal experience, and the skills covered in this book can be helpful for anyone to effectively address problematic anxiety. However, there are certain things you might be dealing with that would make this book an especially good fit. Go through the list of issues below and check off ones that apply to you.

☐ I worry about things more than I would like to.

☐ I have difficulty sleeping because of anxious thoughts.

☐ I experience a lot of physical tension (in my shoulders, neck, and so on).

☐ When I get anxious about something, I often have a hard time stopping or controlling my anxious thoughts.

☐ My anxiety can make it difficult for me to concentrate.

☐ I spend a lot of time thinking about things that could go wrong.

☐ People have told me I'm a "worrier."

☐ I get headaches or muscle aches when I'm stressed.

☐ I have a hard time relaxing.

☐ I get irritable or have a "short fuse" when I'm worrying.

☐ I procrastinate or avoid tasks that make me anxious.

Did you check a lot of boxes? If so, you are absolutely not alone, and this workbook is for you. Even if you checked only a few, if you find yourself distressed by them, this book will likely offer many helpful tools for you. Throughout the book, we'll offer several skills and give you examples of how to apply them to a variety of situations.

You should also know that this book has been written to work both as a stand-alone self-help workbook and as a tool used in conjunction with a therapist. The approach used in this book is based on cognitive behavioral therapy, or CBT, so if you're seeing a therapist familiar with CBT it can be especially helpful to talk with that person about what you're working on and learning here. Even if you're doing a different type of therapy though, this book can be a useful tool for addressing your anxiety.

There are a number of issues that this book isn't designed to address. If you're experiencing suicidal thoughts, feeling severely down and depressed, or drinking alcohol or using other substances in a way that's causing problems, it's important that you get in touch with a mental health professional who can work with you directly on these issues.

Structure of the Workbook

This workbook is divided into seven modules, and each one covers a different skill or set of skills. Each module, or section with the module, includes:

- Informational reading about a concept related to anxiety, including information about how and why the skill works

- Examples of how these concepts and skills can apply to someone struggling with anxiety

- Activities to illustrate the concepts presented

- A review of the key concepts at the end of each section

- Homework exercises for you to monitor your anxiety and practice the skills you've learned

You'll see that this workbook is meant to be very active. That's because you don't learn how to deal with anxiety by simply reading about it! People who effectively address their anxiety do it by practicing! We'll ask you to try new skills and practice different behaviors to break the cycle of anxiety. Because this is a learning process, give yourself plenty of time to practice and absorb what you're learning. We recommend that you complete one module each week. For modules with multiple sections, we suggest one section each week. The only exception is sections I and II of the first module, which you can do together if you'd like. If you follow this schedule, it will take you eleven weeks. Whatever pace you decide to use, we encourage you to plan out when you'll work on each module to keep yourself accountable. We've included a scheduling tool at the end of this section.

Below is a brief outline of what you'll be learning in each module of treatment. These skills form the foundation of cognitive behavioral and mindfulness-based therapies, which research has consistently shown to be the most effective treatments (Carpenter et al. 2018, Hofmann et al. 2010). In addition, the authors of this book have seen these strategies dramatically change the lives of hundreds of patients, so you're getting some of the best tools out there.

- **Module 1: Planning Your Journey:** In this module, you'll set goals for yourself, consider your motivations for addressing anxiety, learn how to better understand your anxiety, and learn about the causes of anxiety.

- **Module 2: Mindful Relaxation:** This is when you learn your first anxiety-reduction skills. This module will teach you two relaxation techniques: progressive muscle relaxation and mindful breathing.

- **Module 3: Rethinking Thoughts:** In this module, you'll learn how habitual patterns of thinking can increase anxiety and how to identify thinking traps. We'll teach you methods for challenging unhelpful, anxious thoughts.

- **Module 4: Worries About Worries:** Here you'll learn to identify how your beliefs about worry and anxiety can escalate anxiety. You'll also practice a mindfulness skill that helps you relate differently to your anxious thoughts.

- **Module 5: Facing Feared Scenarios and Images:** This module will teach you how to face feared situations. Some of these situations may be based in reality, while others may only be in your imagination. Whatever the source, this technique can help you overcome your anxiety.

- **Module 6: Changing Behaviors:** This module involves identifying the behaviors that are maintaining your anxiety. We'll show you how to create a plan for actively changing these behaviors.

- **Module 7: Progress on Goals and Relapse Prevention:** You'll conclude by reviewing the progress you've made toward your goals. You'll also learn how to maintain and build upon the changes you've made.

The following chart lists some of the key questions that will be addressed in each of the modules. Some of these questions are probably more relevant for you than others, and there is a good chance the modules that address those questions will help you the most. However, we encourage you to still go through all modules first, and then you can go back and spend more time on the ones that are most beneficial to you.

Module	Will help you with the following questions...
Module 1: Planning Your Journey	• What are your goals? • Is anxiety a problem for you? • Are you ready to tackle it?
Module 2: Mindful Relaxation	• Are you overly tense? • Do you have trouble relaxing? • Do you have trouble breathing? • Do you have trouble concentrating and being in the present moment?
Module 3: Rethinking Thoughts	• Do you have a lot of automatic negative thoughts? • Do you sometimes make a bigger deal out of things than you need to? • Do you often assume the worst?
Module 4: Worries About Worries	• Does it feel like worrying can help prevent bad outcomes? • Do you worry about the consequences of worrying? • Is it hard for you to shift your attention away from your negative thoughts?
Module 5: Facing Feared Scenarios and Images	• Is there anything that you do or don't do that prevents you from facing your fear? • Are there any images or situations that you fear a lot and that you tend to avoid? • How can you overcome your avoidance?
Module 6: Changing Behaviors	• What worry-driven behaviors end up making your anxiety worse? • How can you identify and change these behaviors?
Module 7: Progress on Goals and Relapse Prevention	• In what areas have you made progress? • How can you keep up the good work? • What areas need further improvement?

Making the Most of the Workbook

As you move through this workbook, follow these guiding principles to get as much benefit as possible:

1. **Consistent practice:** Reading through a module in this workbook probably won't take you much more than hour. However, there are 168 hours in a week, and what you do in those other 167 hours each week will impact your anxiety more than the hour you spend reading this book. So that means practice, practice, practice. Early on, "practicing" will largely mean monitoring and tracking your anxiety, but as you go through the workbook you'll be exposed to more and more skills. The more you practice them, the more helpful they will become. You probably have a lot of things going on in your life, and making enough time for the exercises in this book will be difficult given your other commitments. But try to think of the time as an investment. Putting the time in now can free up a lot of time and energy down the road when you get to the place where you are better able to manage your anxiety.

2. **Be patient:** Anxiety often develops as a result of many years of thinking and behaving in a particular way. That doesn't mean it can't be changed, but it takes time to change those habits. Anticipate frustration, but be patient with yourself if you find that some skills don't immediately work. Staying patient and committed, even when the gains feel small at first, is key to changing your anxiety.

3. **Use social support:** Getting support from others as you go through this book can go a long way toward maximizing your benefits. Other people can provide extra motivation or offer ideas about difficult concepts or exercises. Sometimes, simply having another perspective might help you see your anxiety differently.

4. **Watch out for perfectionism:** People who experience a lot of anxiety often have a strong urge to do things perfectly. While striving for excellence is always a praiseworthy goal, perfectionism can cause problems when it makes people lose sight of what is most important about what they're working on or, even worse, leads people to avoid doing something important because they're worried they can't do it perfectly. Ultimately, there is no perfect way to do the skills presented in this book, so just try your best!

5. **Make it work for you:** This book will present skills and strategies developed and tested by experts in the treatment of anxiety disorders, but you are the expert on your own life. There is no cookie-cutter approach to transforming your anxious mind, so use the

material in this book in the way that works best for you. We encourage you to give every skill in the book an honest shot, but anticipate that some skills will work better for you than others. There are also a host of materials available for download at the website for this book: http://www.newharbinger.com/44529.

Your Workbook Companions

Throughout this workbook, you'll hear about the experiences of three individuals who also experience anxiety, with the hope that it helps you deepen your understanding of the material. Although these characters are fictional, the difficulties they experience are common among individuals who seek treatment for anxiety. Read about these characters below and see if you relate to any of their challenges.

Jill

Jill is in her early thirties and has a job at a consulting firm. She works a lot; she's often one of the first to arrive and the last to leave the office, and she regularly does work on the weekends even though most of her colleagues don't. In many ways, this hard work has been rewarded throughout her life. She always did well in school, and has steadily worked her way up through the firm. Despite her track record, she's constantly worried she's underperforming or not doing enough. She will spend hours going over a presentation in meticulous detail, making relatively unimportant changes, and going back and forth about the best way to do things. She always has her work phone on hand, is constantly checking her email, and feels the need to respond immediately to anything work related, even late at night. Over the last several years, her anxiety about work has started causing problems in her personal life. She avoids making plans with friends because she's busy with work, and she often cancels on friends at the last minute because something comes up. When she does see them, her mind is on her work, to the point where she has difficulty enjoying herself. On top of this, she's anxious about the fact that she's still single. She wants a relationship, but has largely avoided dating the last few years because of how busy she is. The idea of finding a partner and fitting a relationship into her busy work schedule feels overwhelming.

Elijah

Elijah is a graduate student in his mid-twenties, and has significant difficulties with procrastination. He constantly puts off schoolwork because it stresses him out, and when he does work on an assignment, he tends to get extremely anxious about whether he's doing a good job, leading to further avoidance. Although he did quite well in school as an undergraduate, he's received some severe criticism of his work as a graduate student, and now feels as if he has to turn in a perfect product. His fear of doing a poor job and his ensuing procrastination have caused him to fail some classes, and he's going to have to pay for an extra semester of courses in order to graduate. As a result, Elijah is facing financial problems. He has debt from student loans and credit cards. Thinking about how he's going to pay them off causes him to feel panicky, so his mail remains unopened for months, further worsening his financial problems. He lives with his girlfriend, who tries to be supportive, but his anxiety often causes him to be highly irritable toward her, and their relationship has been plagued by arguments the last several months. He has difficulty sleeping. He tosses and turns all night, and feels like his mind won't "shut off." He then feels fatigued throughout the day, and has difficulty concentrating on his work and classes.

Sofia

Sofia is in her late fifties, is married, and has sixteen- and nineteen-year-old sons. She worries constantly about the safety and well-being of her children, particularly her elder son, who just went off to college. She calls and texts her children multiple times each day. If they don't respond, she assumes the worst, which usually involves them being in a terrible accident. She realizes her worries are irrational, but that doesn't quell her intense anxiety. Sofia also feels easily overwhelmed by minor things like getting places on time or completing errands. She feels like she never has enough time to get things done, and she gets worked up if she thinks there is a possibility she will be late to something, even though she's always extremely early. She hasn't worked for years due to the stress. Because of her anxiety, Sofia often experiences intense headaches and neck pain, which trigger further worry about her mental and physical health. She's had a series of medical procedures over the last few years, and she worries that her body is deteriorating because of how much she worries. She spends a lot of time researching possible physical ailments she might be suffering from on the Internet, and has scheduled numerous doctors' appointments because she was convinced she had a brain tumor or other serious medical issue.

You'll hear much more about Jill, Elijah, and Sofia throughout this book. As you learn more about yourself, you'll also get a chance to better understand how their anxiety works, and how it can be helped by the strategies you'll be learning.

Planning and Tracking Your Progress

Use the scheduler on the next page to plan when you'll complete each section of the workbook, and to track your progress (also available at http://www.newharbinger.com/44529).

Section Review: Key Points

- Congratulations on starting this workbook! Acknowledging your anxiety is the first step toward learning to better manage it.

- This book can help you address anxious worries that are difficult to control and the associated problems like muscle tension, difficulty sleeping, irritability, and difficulty concentrating.

- This workbook is intended to be used actively. To make the most of it, practice the techniques you learn consistently, be patient, use social support, watch out for perfectionism, and figure out how to make these techniques work best for you.

Module	Planned Date of Completion	Date Completed
Introduction: How to Use This Workbook		

Module 1: Planning Your Journey
    Section I: Goal Setting and Motivation
    Section II: The Nature of Anxiety and Worries
    Section III: How Anxiety Attacks		

Module 2: Mindful Relaxation		

Module 3: Rethinking Thoughts
    Section I: Probability Overestimation
    Section II: Catastrophizing		

Module 4: Worries About Worries
    Section I: Detached Awareness
    Section II: Worry Postponement		

Module 5: Facing Feared Scenarios and Images		
Module 6: Changing Behaviors		
Module 7: Progress on Goals and Relapse Prevention		

Planning Your Journey

The three sections of this first module will help paint a picture of what your journey toward reducing your anxiety will look like. First, you'll think about what you actually want to change about your life and why. Second, you'll learn what exactly anxiety and worry are, and will start monitoring the ways they affect your life. Third, you'll learn about the different components of anxiety, and how they interact to create a vicious cycle. By the end of this module, you'll have the foundational knowledge you need to start making some real changes.

SECTION I

Goal Setting and Motivation

Hopefully you're feeling some excitement and optimism about using this workbook to reduce the impact that anxiety has on your life. However, it's important to acknowledge that change is difficult. You are likely reading this book because you've formed patterns of anxious thinking and behaving that have developed for some time. Perhaps some of these habits even feel comfortable and easy, at least in comparison to the alternative. Change can also be intimidating because it takes sustained work and effort. For this reason, it can be helpful to think about your motivation for addressing anxiety, and be honest with yourself about the likely challenges. This serves as an explicit reminder of what reducing your anxiety can do for you, and it can help you anticipate possible barriers to actually making that change.

To illustrate this, let's look at Sofia's worksheet, where she listed the pros and cons of *changing*, as well as the pros and cons of *staying the same*.

Pros of Changing	Cons of Changing
• Fewer headaches and neck pain • Wouldn't bother my kids so much • If I'm less anxious, maybe I could go back to work • It would be nice to be able to relax and enjoy myself a little more	• I've lived with anxiety all my life, I don't know who I'd be without anxiety • I'm afraid of trying and failing • Already busy and stressed, not sure I have time

Pros of Staying the Same	Cons of Staying the Same
• It's familiar • My anxiety about others makes me a caring person, and I don't want to give that up	• Being anxious all the time is exhausting • I'll continue to spend a lot of my time worrying • My anxiety will continue to affect my physical health

You can see that Sofia has many good reasons for changing, and there are some significant costs of not doing anything about her anxiety. At the same time, she will face challenges if she decides to make a change. Like Sofia, many people feel that anxiety is a part of their identity and contributes to positive qualities, such as being caring. Moreover, the uncertainty of change can be unsettling. To use the popular idiom, anxiety is *the devil you know*. It's not fun, but at least it's familiar. In addition, Sofia's fear of failure is also common. Sometimes people worry that if they do something about their anxiety and it doesn't work, then it means they'll be anxious forever, which would be even worse. Although you can probably see why the logic behind this is problematic, the worry about failure and associated feelings of helplessness are quite typical for people with anxiety.

Thinking About Change

In spite of all these possible costs and challenges, ask yourself, "Does change seem like it would be worth it for Sofia?" Then ask yourself: "Why do I want to work on my anxiety?" Fill out the boxes below to identify your own reasons for change and the difficulties you anticipate. Try to come up with as many things as you can, even if they seem minor or insignificant. This worksheet is available http at://www.newharbinger.com/44529.

Pros of Changing	Cons of Changing

Pros of Staying the Same	Cons of Staying the Same

Review what you wrote above. Does change seem worth it? Write why or why not below.

_____

_____

_____

_____

Hopefully at this point, you feel like the pros outweigh the cons, but if you are ambivalent about change, know that this is normal, too. The reason for this exercise is first for you to realize all the reasons you have for wanting to change. But it's also good to expect that some things might get in the way. As you proceed through the workbook, we hope you'll realize that some of the cons of changing aren't such a concern after all. For instance, we'll talk about how changing your anxiety doesn't mean changing who you are. You'll also get the opportunity to see for yourself whether the time you invest in practicing the skills in this book pays off (we're confident it will!), even if it's hard to fit into a busy life. It's normal for motivation to wax and wane and for doubts to come up, but don't use that as a reason to abandon your efforts. Instead, come back to what you wrote above and remind yourself of your important reasons for change.

Goal Setting

Another helpful way to motivate yourself toward change is to set goals. Simply writing your goals can increase how hard you work toward them and thereby increase the likelihood of achieving them (Webb and Sheeran 2006). The type of goals you set for yourself, however, will impact how helpful goal setting is. For instance, you might have the following goal for yourself:

I don't want to feel anxious.

If that's what you're hoping for, you're reading the right book! But, there are problems with stating a goal like this. Research shows that the most effective goals are 1) specific and concrete, and 2) challenging but realistic (Locke and Latham 2002). The goal above is certainly not very specific. For example, in what types of situations do you not want to feel anxious? Are there certain things that trigger your anxiety that you'd particularly like to work on? What would it look like to not feel anxious? Or put another way, what would tangibly be different about your life if you weren't so anxious? These sorts of questions can help you make more concrete goals by identifying the specific aspects of your life that you'd like to change. By creating such specific goals, you'll be better able to evaluate whether you've reached them or not. A good goal is something that you could check off a list after accomplishing it.

The second problem with the goal listed above is that it's not very realistic, which can make it easy to lose motivation. While never experiencing anxiety might sound nice, that's not something that anyone is likely to achieve (nor is it necessarily desirable, as we'll talk about in the next section). So instead of thinking about getting rid of anxiety altogether, try to think about some realistic, achievable outcomes for what your life would look like if anxiety were less interfering.

To see what this looks like, review the goals listed by Jill, Elijah, and Sofia. You can see that they start off a bit more general, but are followed up by specific, observable, and attainable descriptions of what reaching their broader goals would look like.

Jill

Goal: Create a healthier balance between work and personal life

What would that look like? How would you know when you've gotten there? Be specific and concrete!

1. Go out with friends at least once per week

2. Don't check my work phone while socializing or relaxing

3. Create an online dating profile and go on at least three dates

4. Leave work in time for an evening yoga class at least twice per week

Notice that Jill's goal isn't specifically about anxiety. Rather, it's about something she wants to be different in her life, but anxiety is getting in the way of accomplishing that. This can be helpful because thinking about what life could be like if anxiety weren't so interfering can be a stronger motivator than just not feeling anxious in certain situations.

Elijah

Goal: Stop procrastinating so much and get on top of my schoolwork

What would that look like? How would you know when you've gotten there? Be specific and concrete!

1. Pass all my classes for the upcoming semester

2. Do at least 30 minutes of schoolwork every weekday evening

3. Reduce anxiety about having my assignments criticized so that I can get them done on time

4. Meet and talk with my professors twice per semester

Elijah's goal starts out as something fairly general ("get on top my schoolwork"), but he narrows it down to much more concrete goals. He also includes a goal (#3) about reducing anxiety, but it's very specific to a particular situation, and he clarifies what he'd like to be able to accomplish as a result (getting assignments done on time). He also follows that up with a specific strategy he could use to help that anxiety.

Sofia

Goal: Prevent minor stressors from turning into major anxiety attacks

What would that look like? How would you know when you've gotten there? Be specific and concrete!

1. Notice my anxiety earlier so I can prevent my emotions from escalating

2. Use relaxation strategies to calm my nerves

3. Prioritize tasks on a to-do list when I'm feeling like I have too much to do

4. Limit the number of times I check in with my kids to one call or text per day

If you're someone like Sofia who worries a lot about a wide variety of little things in your day-to-day life, it can be more challenging to come up with specific goals. Making goals about how you notice and respond to these minor stressors can be helpful.

Now that you've seen some examples, start thinking about your own goals, and write them in the space below. This can be challenging, so take your time. Consider the areas where anxiety is most distressing and identify what you'd like to be doing in your life if anxiety were less interfering. Then get specific and concrete about what it would take to get there. Don't be afraid to revisit this section as you move through the workbook and add additional goals. This worksheet is available at http://www.newharbinger.com/44529.

Goal-Setting Worksheet

Goal #1: _____

What would that look like? How would you know when you've gotten there? Be specific and concrete!

1. _____

   _____

2. _____

   _____

3. _____

   _____

4. _____

   _____

5. _____

   _____

Goal #2: _____

What would that look like? How would you know when you've gotten there? Be specific and concrete!

1. _____

   _____

2. _____

   _____

3. _____

   _____

4. _____

   _____

5. _____

   _____

Goal #3: _____

What would that look like? How would you know when you've gotten there? Be specific and concrete!

1. _____

   _____

2. _____

   _____

3. _____

   _____

4. _____

   _____

5. _____

   _____

Section Review: Key Points

- Changing how you respond to anxiety can be difficult, so revisit the benefits of change and the costs of staying the same. There are usually a lot of really good reasons for you to work on your anxiety!

- It's natural to have mixed feelings, or ambivalence, about change. Don't let that throw you off. Be prepared for the possible barriers and keep at it!

- To stay motivated, write down concrete, observable, and attainable goals and identify what you'd like to accomplish by working on your anxiety. Revisit your goals frequently as you progress through this book.

Home Practice

- **Reflection:** Reflect on your reasons for change and write down your goals.

The Nature of Anxiety and Worries

Now that you're oriented to the workbook and have set some goals, it's time to answer the question: what exactly is anxiety? This might feel like a basic question, but defining anxiety, recognizing why it exists, and understanding how it becomes problematic will establish a framework for learning out how best to intervene. Let's start with the basics.

The Purpose of Anxiety

Anxiety is a universally experienced emotion that alerts us to possible danger. It's like our body's alarm system and is essential for our survival. For example, anxiety directs us to jump out of the way if a car is driving at us, back off if we see a poisonous snake, or avoid a swim in the ocean if there is a storm. In extreme cases, anxiety helps us avoid life-threatening situations. In less extreme scenarios, anxiety prompts us to prepare for a threat to something we care about. For instance, it can encourage us to start preparing ahead of time for a presentation we want to do well on or to check in with a family member who was supposed to be home an hour ago. Because anxiety serves a very important function, our goal isn't to eliminate anxiety altogether. Rather, we want to be able to distinguish between when anxiety is helping us and when it's hurting us.

What Makes Anxiety Problematic?

Anxiety is problematic when one or both of the following are true: 1) it interferes with your functioning or 2) it causes more distress than a situation warrants. For an example, let's consider Jill's situation. At times her anxiety is quite helpful because it drives her to work hard to meet deadlines, produce high-quality work, and maintain her employment. When the anxiety gets more intense, however, she stays too late at work trying to make sure everything is perfect, has difficulty concentrating or making decisions, which causes careless mistakes, and has trouble sleeping because she's worrying about what she has to do the next day. This all comes at the expense of her social life. Jill's anxiety moves from adaptive to problematic because it prevents her from doing things that are important to her (seeing her friends) and interferes with the quality of her work.

For Sofia, her anxiety about her children's well-being encourages her to engage in behavior reflective of a caring and attentive mother. However, when she texts her elder son who is away at college and doesn't hear back for a couple of hours, she starts envisioning that something awful has happened. She begins texting him excessively, which causes him to become irritated with her. Her anxiety response is problematic because the situation starts causing much more distress than is warranted and it strains the relationship.

On the next page we've listed some common areas in which anxiety causes interference or leads to severe distress. Take a few minutes to identify the ways in which anxiety has become problematic for you, and write them down in the space provided.

Generalized Anxiety Disorder: What Is It, and Do I Have It?

Generalized anxiety disorder, or GAD for short, is one type of anxiety disorder that includes a combination of symptoms that make up one of the most common forms of problematic anxiety. While the exact diagnostic criteria are more detailed than this, for our purposes there are two key features of GAD:

1.   Excessive worry that feels uncontrollable

2.   High physical tension

Let's start by talking about worry. *Worry is an unhelpful thinking response to a potential problem.* When people worry, they tend to focus on possible bad outcomes or things that could go wrong. They also might think about what they should do about a situation, but they're *not actually doing anything or actually working toward a solution.* Worry is kind of like a broken record: you keep spinning the same thoughts over and over again in your mind, but you aren't moving forward. For individuals with GAD, worry is very difficult to control, so once your mind starts worrying, it doesn't really stop. In fact, it often escalates, starting with what might be a relatively minor negative outcome and then jumping to an increasingly serious and dire set of concerns that begin to feel like very legitimate possibilities. Commonly, we hear people say that their mind is "constantly racing" or that their thoughts are "difficult to shut off."

Areas of Interference and Distress from Anxiety

Work or School _____

_____

_____

Family _____

_____

_____

Social Life _____

_____

_____

Physical Health _____

_____

_____

Other _____

_____

_____

Worry also has a twin named rumination, which involves thinking over and over about something negative that happened *in the past*. The difference is that worry is always about the future. Worry and rumination do frequently come hand in hand—ruminating about a mistake in the past causes you to worry about making the same mistake in the future—and both are unproductive.

The second primary symptom of GAD is high physical tension. Commonly, this manifests as muscle tension and tension headaches, but tension can also lead to gastrointestinal distress, nausea, fatigue, muscle aches and pains, or restlessness. When your body is persistently tense, it also makes it difficult to sleep, concentrate, or make decisions, and can make you feel keyed up, on edge, and irritable. Sometimes these symptoms clearly coincide with acute periods of heightened anxiety, such as feeling nauseous and having difficulty concentrating just before a big presentation. Many of these symptoms, however, are the result of built-up tension from chronic stress and worry.

So, do you have GAD? Ultimately that question should be answered by a mental health professional through a clinical interview, but if excessive worry and high levels of physical tension are consistently present in your life, you could be experiencing GAD. In reality, what is most important isn't whether you meet the criteria for GAD, but what you wrote down in the section above about the interference and distress that anxiety causes for you. If worry and physical tension are causing impairment in your life, then doing something about your anxiety is warranted, so keep reading!

Why Do I Have So Much Anxiety?

As people begin to learn more about anxiety, a common question arises: why is this such a problem for me? You probably know people in your life who never seem fazed by anything, or even if they do get anxious at times, it doesn't turn into a big ordeal. So what makes you different? We'll use the following formula to understand this better.

Problematic Anxiety = Vulnerability + Stress

By vulnerability, we mean a wide array of biological, developmental, and personality factors that cause someone to be more susceptible to developing high levels of anxiety. Vulnerabilities alone don't cause problems, but under certain conditions, they place certain people at higher risk for problematic anxiety. We've listed common vulnerability factors below. Read through the list and check off those that are relevant for you as you consider your own personal vulnerabilities. This list isn't exhaustive, so add any others that you think of at the bottom.

Vulnerability Factors for Anxiety

☐ Family members with significant anxiety or other mental health issues (genetics)

☐ Parents or other caregivers growing up were anxious, and modeled anxious behavior

☐ Unstable life circumstances growing up (poverty, instability, abuse)

☐ Perfectionism

☐ Having high standards

☐ Emotional sensitivity (feeling emotions more strongly, being sensitive)

☐ Difficulty tolerating uncertainty

☐ High levels of conscientiousness

☐ Neuroticism

☐ Aversion to risk

☐ Fear of failure

☐ Other: _____

☐ Other: _____

You might notice that some of these characteristics are not necessarily negative. High standards and perfectionism can drive you to excel at things. Emotionally sensitive people are often caring and empathic. Conscientiousness involves being responsible and doing things thoroughly and carefully. Changing your anxiety won't mean giving up these traits altogether. Rather, these are characteristics that in certain circumstances, such as under high levels of stress, can end up causing problematic levels of anxiety. We want to reduce the extent to which these factors drive your anxiety by helping you learn some different ways of thinking and behaving in response to stress.

The second part of our formula above that can lead to problematic anxiety is stress. Here, we define stress broadly as any disruptions to the status quo. Stress can be acute (like a deadline or sudden necessary purchase) or chronic (like a highly demanding job or ongoing financial problems). Stress can be anticipated (like an upcoming doctor's appointment) or unanticipated (suddenly learning about a loved one's cancer diagnosis). Stress can also be associated with a positive event (like getting married or starting a new school program) or a negative one (like getting divorced or failing out of school). Often, during periods of more intense stress, anxiety increases. Sofia, for instance, has a history of medical problems. Although there aren't any issues currently, the stress of dealing with them in the past created a lot of anxiety for her, and she continues to be worried about something like that happening again. For Elijah, the transition to graduate school was a major stressor. He always did well in his undergraduate classes and was able to get away with procrastinating because the assignments weren't as difficult for him. Expectations in graduate school are higher now, both from his professors and from himself, creating a much greater susceptibility to high levels of anxiety.

Think about the stressors that may have contributed to your anxiety in the past, and about those that are in your life now, and write them in the spaces below. Remember that a stressor doesn't have to be monumental or catastrophic to affect your anxiety. For example, having two teenage children is a regular stressor for Sofia, whereas simply having friends in the context of a busy job is a stressor for Jill.

Stressors Contributing to Anxiety

Stressors from my past:

- _____
- _____
- _____
- _____

Current stressors:

- _____
- _____
- _____
- _____
- _____

Finally, to understand why your anxiety has become a problem, consider how vulnerability factors interact with your stressors. For Elijah, high expectations from his professors, the difficulty of his graduate work, and criticism he's received on his past assignments naturally cause stress. The fact that he's highly perfectionistic, however, exacerbates that stress and leads to constant procrastination (because avoiding is easier than dealing with the anxiety of creating a perfect product). Review the vulnerability and stressor lists above, and notice how vulnerabilities and stressors interact for you.

You may think that to address problematic anxiety, you need to change the elements of the equation. However, your vulnerability factors are already part of who you are, and you're not going to try and completely change that. And while you can try hard to reduce the stressors you experience, you can't control everything that happens, making stress an inevitable part of life. Plus, focusing too much on reducing stress can come at the expense of other things you value (for example, Sofia avoids going back to work because she thinks it will be too stressful). Instead, you are going to address how you characteristically *respond* to stress. To do this, let's return to the concept of worry.

Returning to Worry: Worry vs. Problem Solving

Recall that worry is a problematic thinking response that arises in the context of a possible problem. It stands in contrast to problem solving, which involves taking active steps toward addressing a situation. Worry keeps us in our head trying to think our way toward addressing a problem, but it isn't goal directed or productive. Remember the broken record analogy? Worry doesn't progress us forward.

For example, Elijah often worries about what his professor will think about his work when he's trying to write a paper. He spends a lot of time thinking about what he's written, whether it's adequate, whether he might have missed something the professor said in class, and what will happen if he gets a bad grade on the paper. This is a clear worry cycle, because Elijah is mulling over what might happen and isn't making any progress on the paper. Problem solving in this situation could be something like scheduling a time to talk with the professor about the paper, having a classmate read over his work, or committing to write for a 30-minute chunk of time each day. These things are not guaranteed to work, but they give Elijah a chance to address his problem, and just as importantly, these actions interrupt the worry cycle.

To clarify the distinction between worry and problem solving, read through examples 1 and 2 in the chart below. Then for examples 3 and 4, try to identify what worrying and problem solving might look like in the example situations, and write it in the empty boxes. Then, fill in boxes 5 and 6 with situations that trigger worry for you, and identify what worrying and problem solving might look like in those cases.

There are a number of reasonable things you could have put down for situations 3 and 4, but in case you had any trouble, in situation 3, Jill's worrying might have involved spending a lot of time thinking about how she's letting her friend down or upsetting her boss, whereas problem solving could be asking for a one-day extension on the report, letting her boss know she'll respond to the emails tomorrow, or asking her friend if they can meet up 30 minutes later. For situation 4, worry might have driven you to continually wonder whether you had done something wrong and ruined your friendship, whereas problem solving could have been as simple as asking your friend if she was offended and preparing an apology.

Of course, it's easier to think of solutions to a problem when you're removed from it, and it's harder to problem solve when you're feeling intense anxiety. The primary purpose of this exercise isn't to test your problem-solving abilities, but rather to help you clarify the difference between worrying and problem solving. If you can make that distinction, you'll be much better prepared to recognize when you're worrying. Improving this ability is critical, because identifying worry is one of the first steps toward being able to change it.

Self-Monitoring

As mentioned earlier, being able to observe when you are worrying is an important part of reducing your anxiety. So, we'll ask you to do some self-monitoring of anxiety over the next week. You might be thinking, "I already know I'm anxious, why do I need to keep track of it?" but there are a number of reasons why this can be quite helpful:

1. You'll become more aware of when you worry, what you worry about, what your primary triggers are, and just how often it happens. It's not uncommon for people to realize they worry much more than they realized.

2. Tracking your anxiety, when you do it *in the moment,* can actually help interrupt the worry process. Observing, monitoring, and understanding your anxiety is a step toward problem solving.

3. Monitoring your anxiety can help you keep track of your progress as you move through this book.

Situation	Worrying	Problem Solving
1. Elijah is trying to fall asleep but thoughts about his financial situation keep popping up.	Think over and over again about his debt and how long it's going to take to pay off	Schedule a time to look at his bills and start to make a financial plan
2. Sofia had a hectic day and isn't going to have time to make the dinner she planned for some guests.	Think about how disappointed her guests are likely to be, and how it's going to ruin the evening	Let the guests know the change of plans for the menu, and pick up some dessert to make up for it
3. Jill has a report that's due by the end of the day, several unanswered emails from her boss, and she's trying to leave work by 6 p.m. to meet up with a friend.		
4. You said something that may have offended a friend of yours, as she left the party right after you said it and she hasn't spoken to you in two weeks.		
5.		
6.		

Rating Your Anxiety

As part of self-monitoring, you'll be rating the intensity of your anxiety using the subjective units of distress scale, or SUDS for short. SUDS are rated on a 0 to 100 scale, and we've included some anchors on this diagram to help you make your ratings. We'll reference SUDS ratings throughout this book and we'll ask you to record your SUDS for various exercises to help you monitor your anxiety.

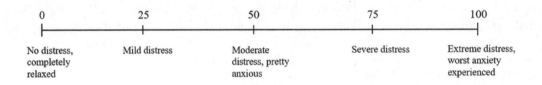

Figure 1.1. *Subjective Units of Distress Scale (SUDS)*

On the next pages you'll see the self-monitoring form you'll be using this week, along with more details on how to complete it.

Self-Monitoring Form

Date and Time	Worry Thought	Time Spent Worrying	SUDS (0–100)
August 24, 11:00 p.m.	[Elijah] If I don't get an A on this paper, I'll never graduate.	1 hour	70

Section Review: Key Points

- Anxiety is a universal emotion that alerts us to the possibility of danger, but it becomes problematic when it starts interfering with our functioning or causing excessive distress.

- Problematic anxiety results from a combination of vulnerability factors (genetics, how you were raised, personality characteristics) and stress.

- Generalized anxiety disorder has two primary components: excessive worry that feels uncontrollable and physical tension (muscle tension, difficulty concentrating, irritability, sleeplessness, fatigue).

- Worry is an unhelpful thinking response to a potential problem that makes anxiety worse. Problem solving is the adaptive alternative to worry and involves taking active steps toward a solution.

Home Practice

- **Self-Monitoring:** Complete the monitoring form below, logging at least one worry thought per day. You can do this as thoughts come up during the day or at the end of day as a reflection. If you don't have your form with you, record your worries on your phone or elsewhere, and then log them in later. However you go about it, the most important thing is to self-monitor consistently and *in the moment*. This worksheet is available at http://www.newharbinger.com/44529.

How Anxiety Attacks

Elijah finally sits down on Sunday evening to write his term paper, which is due on Tuesday. He meant to start working first thing that morning, but the day got away from him. He wasn't able to fall asleep until really late last night, so he let himself sleep in, and then had a leisurely brunch with his girlfriend, decided to do some cleaning around the house, and got some overdue laundry and grocery shopping done. He even spent an hour organizing his desk so he had a pristine working space. The whole day he knew in the back of his mind that he should be working, but he justified the delays by saying he was at least getting something done. Plus, every time he thought about writing the paper, he felt a pit in his stomach, which made him want to look for something else "productive" to do to distract himself. As he opens up his computer at eight o'clock that night and stares at the blank page, the pit in his stomach is still there, except now it's even worse. He thinks about how much he has to write in the next day and a half, how he got a C on the last two papers in this class because he turned them in late, and how he can't get another C or he'll be at risk of being dismissed from his program. He tries writing a few sentences, but he doesn't get very far. The pit in his stomach and all the anxious thoughts running through his head make it hard to concentrate, and he's starting to become jittery and restless. It becomes overwhelming, so he decides to open up the Internet and begins browsing social media. An hour later, he goes back to his paper and sees that he's only written three sentences…

The Anxiety Cycle

In the last section, we talked about how excessive worry and physical tension turn anxiety from a normal and necessary experience into something that causes a lot of problems. In this section, we'll discuss how anxiety can take over and completely derail us from our goals. How exactly did anxiety prevent Elijah from writing more than just a few sentences on his paper nearly twelve hours after he intended to start? What makes it so hard to break out of the anxiety cycle? People often feel helpless to do anything about their anxiety. What gives anxiety that power?

To answer these questions, we first need to break anxiety down into its different component parts. The three components of anxiety are *cognitive*, *physical*, and *behavioral*. Once we see how these components interact, things will begin to make more sense and give us a clearer picture of ways we can intervene. By the end of this section, you'll have a better sense of what anxiety is and how it gets in the way, and a road map for how you can get around it should become clearer.

The Cognitive Component of Anxiety

The cognitive part of anxiety is what goes on in our heads, namely our anxious thoughts. We already covered the cognitive component in the last section when we discussed worry, because worrying produces a lot of anxious thoughts (remember that worry is all in our head). When we're anxious, our thoughts are usually about something that could go wrong ("I'm going to be late!"), or if something has gone wrong, what that's going to mean about the future ("My boss is upset with me, I'm going to get fired!"). Sometimes people have a difficult time identifying what their thoughts are when they're anxious, especially if their anxiety is dominated by physical sensations. Think about it like this: if my anxiety could speak, what would it say? What is it worried about happening? Anxious thoughts often sound like: "What if…?" or "If…happens, then…!"

Below are a few examples of the anxious thoughts that Elijah was likely experiencing when he was trying to write his paper. See if you can come up with a few additional ones to get familiar with identifying the cognitive component of anxiety. Be creative and make things up, or imagine what you'd be thinking in his position.

- I'm going to get a bad grade again.

- I'm so anxious I can't focus.

- _____

- _____

Other thoughts that might have gone through Elijah's head include "I'm going to fail the class and get kicked out of school" or "There's no way I'll be able to get this done in time." You might notice that anxious thoughts tend to be rather extreme. For instance, it's probably not true that that there is no way Elijah won't be able to get his paper done in time. When that's the type of thought that pops up, however, it's easy to see why Elijah would feel so anxious. You'll learn more about different types of thinking patterns, called "thinking traps," and how they contribute to anxiety in Module 3.

For now, read through the list of common anxious thoughts below, checking off any that tend to come up for you, and adding others that you think of.

☐ My friend hasn't texted me back; they are probably upset with me.

☐ I almost certainly have that serious medical condition.

☐ If I don't make this perfect, my boss will think less of me and I could lose my job.

☐ [Someone I care about] is late; something terrible probably happened.

☐ What if I forgot something important? Everything will be ruined!

☐ I'm too anxious to be able to do anything right now.

☐ I'm probably going to do a poor job on this.

☐ I don't know what's going to happen, so I need to be prepared for anything.

☐ _____

☐ _____

☐ _____

☐ _____

The Physical Component of Anxiety

The physical part of anxiety is what goes on in our bodies. Remember that the purpose of anxiety is to alert us to possible danger. One of the ways our brain does this is by changing how our body feels. If we found ourselves in a life-threatening situation—for instance, encountering a poisonous snake—our muscles would instantly tense up, our heart would start pounding to increase blood flow, and our whole nervous system would become activated to help us minimize or avoid the threat by fighting back or running away. This happens in less extreme situations as well, and there are all sorts of ways our bodies attempt to alert us to something possibly going wrong. For Elijah, the pit in his stomach was the most noticeable physical sensation, and he also felt jittery and restless. How does your body feel when you become anxious? Read through the list of common anxiety-related physical sensations and check off the ones that apply to you:

☐ Pounding or racing heart   ☐ Muscle tingling or twitching

☐ Sweating   ☐ Feeling restless or jittery

☐ Clenched jaw   ☐ Gastrointestinal distress

☐ Nausea   ☐ Shaking or trembling

☐ Pit in the stomach   ☐ Shortness of breath

☐ Overheating   ☐ Butterflies in the stomach

☐ Chest pain or tightness   ☐ Muscle tension

☐ Tension headache   ☐ Fatigue

☐ Other: _____

☐ Other: _____

For some people, the physical sensations associated with anxiety are less noticeable or simply aren't as strong. In the upcoming weeks, we'll ask you to start paying more attention to these physical signs of anxiety. You might begin to see that some of them are more present than you realize. After all, many of the symptoms associated with problematic anxiety, such as irritability, sleeplessness, and difficulty concentrating, are partially a result of the accumulation of the physical components of anxiety.

The Behavioral Component of Anxiety

The behavioral part of anxiety refers to what you do as a result of your anxious feelings. Behaviors are typically thought of as involving an action that you can observe (for example, Elijah browses social media or cleans his desk instead of working on his paper). However, behavior can also involve imperceptible or internal action. For example, Elijah might also be sitting in front of his computer just thinking about what will happen if he gets a bad grade on his paper. In that case, we'd say his behavior *is* worry. We can think of worry as a behavior if it describes what someone is doing in response to a situation. Rather than problem solving, which would involve trying out a strategy to make progress on his paper, Elijah is worrying. To be clear, the *actual thoughts* you have when you worry ("I'm going to fail the class") make up the cognitive component of anxiety, but the *act* of worrying is a behavior.

Below is a list of common behaviors associated with anxiety. Check off any that you engage in, and add others to the list if you think of them.

☐ Procrastinating

☐ Seeking reassurance

☐ Venting

☐ Over-preparing or over-researching

☐ Worrying

☐ Checking something over and over

☐ Being extremely cautious

☐ Distracting yourself (with TV, conversation, Internet)

☐ Leaving a situation

☐ Drinking alcohol or using other drugs

☐ Other: _____

☐ Other: _____

Expanding on Behavior: Avoidance

Anxious behaviors are almost always attempts to reduce anxiety. Feeling anxious is unpleasant, so naturally we want to avoid it. Unfortunately, attempts to avoid anxiety are often ineffective, especially in the long term. In fact, avoidance is actually one of the primary reasons why anxiety becomes a persistent problem. To explain how this works, let's first clarify what we mean by avoidance.

Avoidance is anything you do, or don't do, to reduce your anxiety.

Some forms of avoidance are pretty straightforward, like simply avoiding the activity, situation, or thoughts that make you anxious. However, there are a lot of subtle forms of avoidance. For example, avoidance can be partial, like if Jill goes out with her friends but checks her work email throughout dinner. She's not completely avoiding going out with friends, but she's trying to make herself less anxious by constantly checking her email. Other subtle forms of avoidance include things like excessive information gathering (Internet browsing), excessive list making, asking people for reassurance, or mentally reviewing something over and over again. In all these cases, the behavior functions to reduce anxiety, and therefore counts as avoidance.

Sometimes avoidance behaviors *appear* to be productive or helpful, but actually increase anxiety and fail to address the problem. Take over-preparing, for example. Jill's anxiety might drive her to spend an entire weekend working on a presentation for work, which at first glance might seem to be a good thing because it will ensure she does a good job. But if spending more than a couple of hours on the presentation isn't necessary, then the purpose of that behavior becomes more about reducing her anxiety than doing her job well.

Worry is another form of covert avoidance. Like other forms of avoidance, worry can feel productive, or at least necessary, because you're focusing on a potential problem rather than ignoring it or distracting yourself from it. You're not avoiding anxiety altogether when you worry, but it serves the purpose of protecting yourself from the possibility of something bad happening and not being prepared for it. For people who worry a lot, it feels safer to think about everything that could possibly go wrong than to be taken by surprise by an unexpected negative event.

Consider this analogy. Imagine that you are an outfielder in a baseball game. You realize that at some point a ball is going to come your way and you need to be ready to catch it. To prepare, you get in the proper stance, you have your glove ready, and you direct your attention to the pitcher and the batter coming up to the plate so you'll know when the ball is coming. This is certainly better than being totally unprepared for a ball coming your way, which could lead to serious negative consequences. However, chronically worrying is like being braced in a "ready stance" all the time, *even when it isn't a game day.* Although this might help you feel prepared for any possible catastrophe, it comes at a cost of being tense and anxious all the time. In this way, worry attempts to reduce anxiety (making it avoidance), but paradoxically worsens it by contributing to persistent and chronic anxiety.

Short-Term vs. Long-Term Consequences of Avoidance

Avoidance behavior can become habitual and difficult to change. This is because the immediate, short-term consequences of avoidance tend to be highly rewarding. That is, we feel better when we avoid something difficult or anxiety provoking. For example, when Elijah decided to do his laundry instead of working on his paper, he felt an immediate sense of relief because he was no longer thinking about the stress associated with school. Or when Sofia texts her children to make sure they're okay and they respond, she can finally feel calm and at ease knowing that everything is fine. The sense of relief that comes from reducing your anxiety through avoidance behavior is quite powerful, and can lead to the formation of some pretty strong habits.

The major problem with avoidance is that it can also have significant negative consequences, especially in the long term. First, avoidance prevents you from doing things that are important to you. Elijah's avoidance prevents him from spending enough time on his schoolwork. Jill's avoidance prevents her from spending quality time with other people. Sofia's avoidance interferes with her pursuit of employment. In this way, the short-term reward of avoidance gets in the way of longer-term goals.

A second problem of avoidance is that it paradoxically increases anxiety later on. Procrastinating all day only ended up increasing Elijah's anxiety when he went back to work. Jill's avoidance of socializing increases her anxiety about whether her friends are upset with her, and about whether she'll ever find a partner. When Sofia texts her children excessively, it makes her more anxious about their safety than she'd feel if she instead were spending her time and energy engaging in something else she cared about. Avoidance is akin to pushing a problem down the road. Inevitably, it returns, and often even more intensely.

Finally, and perhaps most importantly, avoidance prevents you from learning what happens if you do *not* engage in the avoidance behavior. Every time you engage in avoidance behavior, you teach your body and your brain that you *need* to avoid in order to prevent something bad from happening and to not feel anxious. Avoiding prevents you from even having a chance to learn that your worries might be unrealistic, and that you can actually handle what might happen. To illustrate this further, consider the following story.

Charlie and Fred are walking down the streets of Boston together. At the end of every block, Charlie turns to the nearest building and bangs his head against the wall. Perplexed, Fred eventually asks, "Charlie, why on earth do you keep banging your head against the wall? It must hurt like crazy!" Charlie replies, "Sure it hurts, but it keeps the elephants away." Fred says, "But there are no elephants in Boston." Charlie replies, "See? It works!"

Charlie is convinced that something he's doing (banging his head against a wall) is preventing a bad outcome (elephants coming to Boston), without ever giving himself the chance to see what would happen if he didn't do that, or realizing that such a concern is completely unrealistic in the first place. And in the process, he's actually hurting himself. Avoidance behavior works the same way. For people with problematic anxiety, their anxious concerns are often not entirely realistic, and spending time avoiding them through worry or other means is harmful. It can be difficult to realize that and change your behavior, but you need to give yourself an honest chance of seeing what happens if you behave otherwise. We'll talk much more about how to explicitly address avoidance in Modules 5 and 6. For now, the important thing is to realize the way in which avoidance contributes to the anxiety cycle. As you continue to self-monitor this week, start noticing your avoidance behaviors and how they might be influencing your anxiety in the long term.

How the Components of Anxiety Interact

Let's return now to the three components of anxiety and summarize how they influence each other. It's important to realize that the cognitive, physical, and behavioral components interact to form a vicious cycle of anxiety. Consider figure 1.2, starting with Elijah's situation.

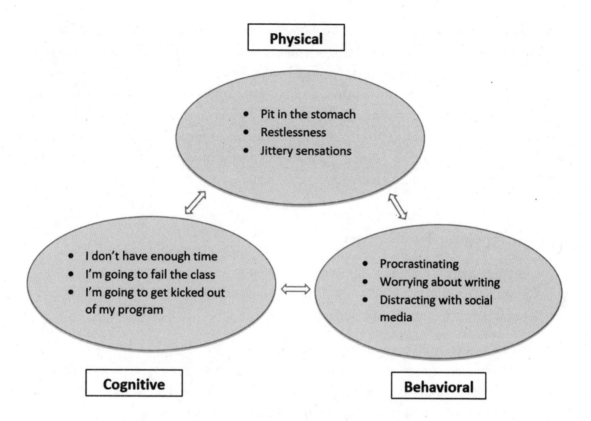

Figure 1.2. *Three Components of Anxiety*

Notice the double-sided arrows going between the three circles, meaning that each component influences the other. Beginning with the physical component, Elijah felt a pit in his stomach when he thought about writing his paper. This caused him to procrastinate (an avoidance behavior) for a good portion of the day. In this way, the physical component of anxiety influenced the behavioral component. After a day of procrastinating, Elijah returned to his paper, and the pit in his stomach got worse. His behavior in turn affected his physical sensations. The procrastination also led to that first anxious thought, "I don't have enough time." In this way, the behavioral component also influenced the cognitive component of anxiety. Elijah's thoughts about not having enough time also increased the intensity of physical sensations (cognitive to physical) and led him to spend his time worrying (remember that worry is a behavior) about what happens if he doesn't do well on the paper (cognitive to behavioral). Finally, we can see how the physical in turn impacted the cognitive. The pit in Elijah's stomach was sending the message back to his brain "this is bad," which exacerbated the intensity of his anxious thoughts.

You can see how tightly connected these components of anxiety are, and how once things get going it can create a cycle of anxiety that's quite difficult to stop. The good news is that the mutual influence of these components of anxiety can work in the opposite direction as well. To start reducing anxiety, you don't need to take on all three components at once. For example, if you can lessen the intensity of your physical sensations when you're anxious, it can help make your worry thoughts and the urge to engage in anxiety-driven behavior a little less powerful. This also means that there are three distinct targets for reducing anxiety. In the rest of this book, you'll learn techniques to address each component of anxiety.

Section Review: Key Points

- Anxiety consists of three components: the cognitive component (your thoughts), the physical component (what you feel in your body), and the behavioral component (what you do in response to your anxiety).

- Anxiety often leads to avoidance behavior, which is anything you *do* or *don't do* to reduce anxiety. Some behaviors like over-preparing, seeking reassurance, or worrying can feel productive, but still count as avoidance if they're done with the primary purpose of reducing anxiety rather than solving an actual problem.

- Avoidance behavior often provides relief in the short term, but in the long term it gets in the way of you reaching your goals, increases anxiety, and prevents you from learning that your worries may be unrealistic.

- The three components of anxiety mutually influence each other, leading to a cycle of anxiety. You'll learn techniques to target each aspect of anxiety. Even working on one component will begin to alleviate the problematic anxiety you experience.

Home Practice

- **Self-Monitoring:** Continue self-monitoring, but this week begin to observe the different aspects of your anxiety. Identify the *thoughts*, *physical sensations*, and *behaviors* involved in your anxiety response, and notice how each component influenced the others. Write down at least one situation each day using the following form (available at http://www.newharbinger.com/44529).

Monitoring the Three Components of Anxiety

Date and Time	Situation	Thoughts	Physical Sensations	Behaviors	SUDS (0–100)
August 31, 8:00 p.m.	[Sofia] Meeting up with a friend after canceling plans before	She's going to be so mad at me. I've probably ruined the friendship.	Increase in heart rate, sweaty palms, butterflies in her stomach	Asked her friend multiple times throughout the night and afterward whether she's mad	80

MODULE 2

Mindful Relaxation

It's been a tough week at work for Jill, and it looks like next week will involve just as many struggles, with last-minute meetings, reports, and yet another presentation in front of her boss. Although she doesn't have to think about it over the weekend, Jill has a hard time not feeling "on edge." Often, her mind will drift off to what's on her plate at work next week rather than relaxing in the present moment. Not only do Jill's worries spiral out of control, but she can feel her anxiety physically as well. Jill always seems to have muscle tension in her neck and upper shoulders. Also, whenever she worries, she tends to pace back and forth or fidget in her seat. She sometimes doesn't even notice how restless she gets. Jill wants to spend her weekend focusing on things she likes, such as getting brunch with her friends and finally finishing that novel for book group that she's been putting off. Her anxiety about the workweek makes her so tense and distracted that she feels like it will be impossible to do any of the fun things she really wants to do. Spending all of her time on her anxiety rather than in the here and now leaves Jill feeling disappointed about her weekend, as if it's all out of her control.

Learning to Relax: Progressive Muscle Relaxation

Does Jill's experience sound familiar? As mentioned in the prior module, some of the most common symptoms associated with anxiety are physical in nature. People who suffer from anxiety and worry often have tension and muscle stiffness that they carry throughout their body. In Jill's case, her excessive tension prevented her from relaxing and enjoying her weekend. Also, being on edge the whole time makes it extremely difficult to focus on the present moment and things going on right now. This can lead to anxiety that spirals out of control, and it can interfere with the things you actually want to do.

So far, you've learned that anxiety has three components: thoughts, physical sensations, and behaviors. To break the vicious cycle of anxiety, it's important to learn strategies that address each one of these domains. The first technique you'll learn targets the physical sensations associated with anxiety, such as muscle tension. Specifically, you'll learn about progressive muscle relaxation (PMR). PMR has a long history, dating back to the early twentieth century, and it's a first-line technique for combatting stress and tension. In brief, PMR is a deep relaxation technique that teaches you how to achieve physical relaxation through a two-step process. First, you apply *tension* to your muscles for a brief amount of time. Second, you *relax* that muscle group for a longer amount of time.

As simple as it is, PMR can be used throughout the body on a variety of muscle groups. The overall goal of PMR is to learn how to relax the whole body at once. Before we get to that, however, it's important to receive instructions on each step.

PMR: The Basics

Before we dive into PMR, it's important to distinguish between two types of applied tension. The first type is called *active tensing*. This type of tension occurs when you are purposefully trying to tense a particular muscle group as hard as you can without hurting yourself. PMR often starts with using active tensing for isolated muscle groups. After practice, it can be used for multiple muscle groups at the same time, and eventually the whole body. In general, active tensing is the standard type of tension you use while practicing PMR. Active tensing often leads to deeper feelings of relaxation.

The second type of tension is called *passive tensing*. Unlike active tensing, passive tensing involves merely noticing whatever tensions already exist in a particular muscle group. That is, you are not purposefully attempting to apply tension. Although active tensing is often preferred because it usually leads to greater relaxation, there might be some circumstances in which you want to consider passive tensing. In particular, passive tensing is often recommended for muscles or regions of your body that have suffered an injury or are in pain. It's important not to cause further injury to any part of your body, which makes passive tensing a worthwhile alternative. With passive tensing, you note the tension that exists in a muscle area and then focus greater efforts on the relaxation phase.

It's important to think about your approach to the relaxation phase. In general, you want to use any type of verbal phrase or mantra that invokes the idea of deep relaxation. This could include concepts such as heaviness, sleepiness, or calmness. Feel free to use whatever is helpful for you. Below we provide a few examples of different phrases that can focus your mind on relaxation.

Relaxation Phrases

- *Relax…*

- *Calm…*

- *Let your muscles feel heavy…*

- *Let your muscles feel like lead weights…*

- *Notice the tension melt away…*

- *Notice yourself feeling calm and rested…*

- *Feel the relaxation deeper and deeper…*

- *Notice the difference between tension and relaxation…*

At this point, please write down whatever phrase you'd like to use below. For the purpose of demonstrating the exercise, we'll tell you to say the word "relax," but you can change this with whatever phrase you prefer.

_____

_____

_____

Also keep in mind that the relaxation phase will always be longer than the tension phase! In general, you should tense your muscles for a relatively short amount of time, and then take a longer period of time to allow yourself to enter into a state of deep relaxation. Don't give in to the temptation to quickly pass over the relaxation phase just to move on to the next muscle group! You'd be selling yourself short of getting the best benefits from PMR. It's important to have patience when it comes to this exercise. If you move too quickly from muscle group to muscle group, you might end up feeling more stressed out! So please, take your time, and allow yourself to experience deep relaxation. There is no rush.

You'll learn two PMR exercises in this module. You'll start with the twelve-muscle-group PMR. Once you have learned this and feel comfortable with it, you'll decrease your PMR exercise to just eight groups (by combining some of the muscle groups). Eventually, you'll have the goal of being able to relax with just one step.

For the PMR exercise, pick a quiet space with a comfortable chair or bed. When positioning yourself, please sit in an upright posture, and make sure you have enough space in front of you to move your arms and legs. Initially, you should choose a place that's not distracting. Make sure to wear loose clothing and take off glasses or contact lenses. The exercise will take about 20 to 30 minutes, so make sure you are able to set aside time for this during the day.

PMR for Twelve Muscle Groups

Now we are ready to begin! Please keep your relaxation phrase (such as "relax") in mind while practicing, and remember not to use active tension on any muscle groups or areas of your body that are injured. Consider skipping that injured muscle or using passive tension for that muscle instead.

1. Close your eyes and relax. Take some deep breaths from your belly as you sit quietly.

2. Produce tension in your lower arms by making fists and pulling up on your wrists so that your wrists nearly touch your shoulders. Focus on the tension (10 seconds). Now release the tension in your lower arms and hands. Let your arms relax with your palms down. Focus your attention on the feeling of relaxation and relax your muscles (50 seconds). Continue to breathe deeply and think the word "relax" with each exhale.

3. Produce tension in your upper arms by leaning forward, pulling your arms back and in to the sides of your body, and trying to touch your elbows behind your back. Focus on the tension (10 seconds). Now release your arms and relax (50 seconds), letting all the tension go. Feel the difference between the tension and the relaxation. As you sit quietly, say the word "relax."

4. Produce tension in your lower legs by flexing your feet up and bringing your toes toward your upper body, trying to touch your toes to your knees. Feel the tension in your feet, ankles, shins, and calves. Focus on the tension (10 seconds). Now release the tension and feel the difference between the tension and the relaxation (50 seconds). As you sit quietly, think the word "relax" with each exhale from your belly.

5. Produce tension in your upper legs by bringing your knees together and lifting your legs off the chair. Focus on the tension in your upper legs (10 seconds). Now, release the tension in your legs and feel the difference between the tension and the relaxation. Focus on the feeling of relaxation (50 seconds). Think the word "relax" as you continue to sit quietly, breathing deeply.

6. Produce tension in your stomach by pulling your stomach tightly in toward your spine. Feel the tension and tightness; focus on that part of your body (10 seconds). Now let your stomach go and relax outward. Feel the comfortable feeling of relaxation (50 seconds), and as you sit quietly, think the word "relax" with each exhale.

7. Produce tension around your chest by taking a deep breath and holding it. Feel the tension in your chest and back. Hold your breath (10 seconds). Now relax and let the air out slowly (50 seconds) and feel the difference between the tension and the relaxation. As you sit quietly, continuing to breathe deeply and think the word "relax."

8. Produce tension in your shoulders by bringing your shoulders up toward your ears. Focus on the tension in your shoulders and neck (10 seconds). Now drop your shoulders; let them droop and relax. Concentrate on the sensation of relaxation (50 seconds). As you sit quietly, think the word "relax."

9. Produce tension around your neck by tilting your chin down and trying to press the back of your neck against the chair or toward the wall behind you. Focus on the tightness around the back of your neck (10 seconds). Now release the tension and concentrate on the relaxation (50 seconds) and feel the difference between the tension and the relaxation. As you sit quietly, think the word "relax" with each deep exhale.

10. Produce tension around your mouth and jaw by clenching your teeth and pushing the corners of your mouth back. Feel the tension in your mouth and jaw (10 seconds). Now release the tension, allowing your mouth to drop open, and concentrate on the difference between the tension and the relaxation (50 seconds). As you sit quietly, think the word "relax."

11. Produce tension around your eyes by tightly squeezing your eyes shut for a few seconds and then release the tension in your eyes. Feel the difference between the tension and the relaxation (50 seconds). As you sit quietly, continuing to breathe deeply from your belly and think the word "relax."

12. Produce tension across your lower forehead by pulling your eyebrows down toward the center of your face and frowning. Focus on the tension in your forehead (10 seconds). Now relax your forehead and feel the difference between the tension and the relaxation (50 seconds). Think the word "relax" with each exhale.

13. Produce tension in your upper forehead by raising your eyebrows to the top of your head. Focus on the pulling sensation and tension across your forehead (10 seconds). Now relax your eyebrows and focus on the difference between the tension and the relaxation. As you sit quietly, think the word "relax."

14. You are fully relaxed. Continue to sit quietly with your eyes closed and breathe deeply from your belly. Count to yourself from one to five, making yourself feel more and more relaxed. One, allow all of the tension to leave your body. Two, feel yourself dropping further and further down into relaxation. Three, you're feeling more and more relaxed. Four, you're feeling quite relaxed. Five, you're feeling completely relaxed. As you're in this relaxed state, focus on all of your muscles being completely comfortable and stress free. As you sit in this state, breathing deeply, think the word "relax" with each deep exhale (2 minutes).

15. Now, focus on counting backward from five and feeling yourself becoming more alert. Five, you're feeling more alert. Four, you're feeling yourself coming out of the relaxation state. Three, you're feeling more awake. Two, you're opening your eyes. One, you're sitting up and feeling completely awake and alert.

As you can see, physical relaxation is just as important as mental relaxation, which is training yourself to move your attention away from worrisome thoughts and back to the physical sensations of tension and relaxation.

After PMR: Reflection

You've now tried PMR for the first time. For many people, it's not only physical relaxation that they feel, but also mental relaxation. If you noticed this as well, then you've just experienced how deep the connection is between your physical feelings and what is going in your mind. Using the chart below, please track what you noticed before and after PMR!

Rating Symptom Intensity Before and After PMR

Before PMR					After PMR				
Anxiety Symptom	Intensity				Anxiety Symptom	Intensity			
	None	Mild	Moderate	Severe		None	Mild	Moderate	Severe
Neck Tension					Neck Tension				
Upper Back Tension					Upper Back Tension				
Lower Back Tension					Lower Back Tension				
Forehead Tension					Forehead Tension				
Arm Tension					Arm Tension				
Leg Tension					Leg Tension				
Restless, Unable to Relax					Restless, Unable to Relax				
On Edge					On Edge				
Worry					Worry				
Rapid or Shallow Breathing					Rapid or Shallow Breathing				

In general, how were you feeling before trying PMR? _____

_____

How do you feel after trying PMR? _____

_____

PMR Practice

Now that you've tried PMR, it's important to continue practicing this technique. Using any technique only one time is usually insufficient to achieve long-lasting results. Sometimes it's hard to do PMR well the first time. If this was your experience, then you aren't alone! It's good to be patient with yourself as you begin to master PMR. People often notice that it takes time to use PMR effectively. We also recommend practicing PMR in less stressful situations first so you get the hang of it, and then build toward using it when you are particularly stressed. You'll see more specific instructions for your PMR practice for the week at the end of the module.

PMR for Eight Muscle Groups

When you've practiced the twelve-muscle-group exercise for a week and you can reach a state of moderate relaxation (at least 50 or greater on a scale of 0 to 100), you can start doing the eight-muscle-group exercise. The ultimate goal is to be able to achieve a relaxation state with just one step (to engage in full body tension and then relaxation). The eight muscle groups you'll be focusing on for this procedure are: 1) arms, both the lower and upper arms together, 2) legs, both the lower and upper legs together, 3) stomach, 4) chest, 5) shoulders, 6) neck, 7) eyes, and 8) forehead (you can do the upper or lower forehead). You'll use the same tensing and relaxing exercises, concentrating on the sensations and the difference between the feelings of tension and relaxation. As you sit quietly, think the word "relax."

If you'd like to follow a script for the eight-muscle-group exercise, go to http://www.newharbinger.com/44529. As before, practice the eight-muscle-group relaxation daily, and track your progress in the chart provided at the end of the module.

Tips for Advanced PMR

So far, you've learned the basics of PMR, and you've experienced firsthand how muscular tension and relaxation can lead to deep physical relaxation. Up to now, we've asked you to practice PMR in a quiet environment that's relatively free from distractions. However, life isn't always so forgiving, and at any moment, we can be thrown a curveball with little stressors or tasks that demand our attention. To take PMR to the next level, try using it in situations that are distracting or stressful. You can try using PMR at work, during a subway ride, in a busy café, or just about anywhere! It's important to become adept at PMR not only when you have a secluded, quiet environment, but also during the hectic times of your day. So, give PMR a try in a variety of situations to take your mastery to the next level.

Also, another way to make progress with PMR is by using the *combination method* for the different muscle groups. You've already done this in the eight-muscle-group exercise, when you tense and relax both your upper arms and lower arms at the same time. By continuing to combine muscle groups that you tense and relax at the same time, you can eventually get to the point where you use PMR for your whole body in just one step. Getting practice with this is helpful for achieving deep relaxation within a relatively short period of time.

Moving from Physical Relaxation to Mindful Relaxation

So far, you've learned about how to achieve physical relaxation using PMR. But, it's important to realize that relaxation can occur not just at the physical level but also mentally. You may have even noticed that physical relaxation can lead to you feeling calmer mentally. Note, however, that mental relaxation by itself is just as important. We'll now introduce you to *mindfulness* and show you how you can use this skill when relaxing. In essence, mindfulness refers to developing a nonjudgmental and nonreactive awareness of the present moment, giving yourself crucial distance from your thoughts when you don't respond to or evaluate them in any particular way. Furthermore, by grounding your attention in the present moment, you are not letting your mind drift off to worrisome thoughts about the future or troublesome memories from the past.

There are a number of different exercises people can do to get better at mindfulness. One of the most common exercises is called *mindful breathing.* The idea behind mindful breathing is to pay attention to your breathing in a nonjudgmental, nonreactive way. For instance, if you happen to notice a thought pop up in your mind as you are focusing on your breathing, the mindful way of responding to the thought is to just let it be and gently guide your attention back to your breathing. This can be easier said than done sometimes! But with practice, mindfulness can help you build a less judgmental and more peaceful mind. One of the key tricks to mindfulness is be patient and forgiving with yourself when you notice your mind is wandering. A wandering mind is a completely normal response, and it tends to occur more often when you are a novice. Instead of beating yourself up about it, merely note that your mind is wandering and then gently redirect your focus.

Now, let's try your first mindfulness exercise! As mentioned before, the object of your mindful awareness will be your breath. The goal is to just simply focus on your breath and stay grounded in the present moment.

Mindful Breathing Exercise

Find a comfortable and quiet place where you can sit upright on a chair or on a cushion on the floor. You want to have an alert but relaxed posture. This exercise will last for 5 minutes. Once you are seated, set a timer to alert you when the time is up. Then follow the steps below.

1. Close your eyes and relax.

2. Start by inhaling deeply through your mouth for 5 seconds. (Notice how the air feels in your mouth, throat, and lungs as you are inhaling. Let that be the focus of your attention.)

3. After inhaling, hold your breath for 3 seconds.

4. Next, gently exhale through your nostrils for 5 seconds, and mentally count the word "one" as you are exhaling. (Notice how the air feels in your throat and nostrils as you are releasing your breath.)

5. Repeat these steps again (inhale, hold, and exhale), and remember to mentally count the next number ("two," "three," "four") as you exhale. Continue doing this until your 5 minutes is up.

After you've tried your first mindfulness exercise, congratulate yourself! If you noticed any difficulties focusing your mind on your breath, be kind to yourself. Remember that mastering a nonjudgmental, nonreactive awareness takes practice. Please record your initial reactions to the mindfulness exercise below.

How did you feel before the mindfulness exercise?

_____

_____

_____

How do you feel now?

_____

_____

_____

What differences in your thinking do you notice after trying mindful visualization?

_____

_____

_____

If it was hard doing this the first time, then you are not alone. Remember that it's completely normal to find yourself distracted by other sensations or thoughts. When this happens, try to gently remind yourself to return your attention to the breath. Be patient with yourself as you begin to master mindfulness—you'll have plenty of opportunities to practice going forward.

Mindful Cloud Exercise

As you've learned so far, mindfulness can help us develop a calmer and more relaxed mind. Another important benefit of mindfulness is that it can help us counteract our knee-jerk tendency to react to and judge our inner thoughts and experiences. One of the biggest factors that contributes to anxiety is this tendency to impulsively react to feelings and worries. Often, this type of mind-set just leads to a vicious cycle of anxiety consumed by worries and negative reactions. Mindfulness can be an important skill that gives you distance from troublesome thoughts and lets you accept your inner experiences.

The next exercise is the mindful cloud exercise. Just like the last exercise, the main purpose is to achieve present-moment awareness, nonjudgment, and nonreactivity. Rather than focusing on breathing, however, the exercise will use visualization techniques to help you observe your thoughts in a more helpful and less reactive way. The goal is to observe each thought ("Tomorrow's meeting will be a catastrophe"), feeling ("I feel really tense and keyed up"), or emotionally driven behavior ("I want to over-rehearse my part of the presentation tomorrow to avoid messing up") and imagine it being placed on a cloud that slowly floats away.

Find a comfortable and quiet place where you can sit upright on a chair or on a cushion on the floor. You want to have an alert but relaxed posture. This exercise will last for 5 minutes. Once you are seated, set a timer to alert you when the time is up. Then follow the steps below, and try to visualize this scene in as much vividness as you can!

1. Close your eyes and relax.

2. Imagine that you are sitting on a grassy hill overlooking a big open sky. Occasionally, a fluffy cloud emerges from the distance and blows by. Afterward, it slowly drifts off into the horizon until it's no longer visible.

3. Now, take a thought or judgment that's been bothering you lately. Try to visualize the thought as one of those clouds in the sky. Let the thought flow with the breeze, just as the cloud does. Watch it float off into the distance and merge with the other clouds in the background.

4. Remember to just let the cloud float away. Try not to follow the cloud or bring it back. Just stay at your spot on the grassy hill, and observe your thought physically move away from you.

5. Continue this visualization exercise for any other thought or feeling you have. Really try to visualize and feel the physical distance between yourself and the negative thought as it embodies the form of a cloud.

6. If you notice that you are having trouble being nonjudgmental or nonreactive toward a specific thought or "cloud," be patient with yourself.

7. After you finish this visualization for your last thought, slowly take a deep breath and then exhale. Bring your present-moment awareness back to your current environment.

Once you've tried this exercise, you should feel proud of your accomplishment! Difficulties when first trying these exercises are normal, so if you struggled at all, remember to be kind to yourself. Mastering a nonjudgmental, nonreactive stance toward your thoughts takes practice, and you'll get the chance to track your progress in this domain over the next week.

Please record your reactions to the mindful cloud exercise below.

How did you feel before the mindfulness exercise?

_____

_____

_____

How do you feel now?

_____

_____

_____

What differences in your thinking do you notice after trying mindful visualization?

_____

_____

_____

_____

Section Review: Key Points

- Progressive muscle relaxation (PMR) is a technique that can be used to help with the physical sensations associated with anxiety, such as muscle tension.

- The goal of PMR is to create deep physical relaxation by tensing and relaxing your muscles. You may notice that creating physical relaxation influences mental relaxation.

- Another technique to target mental relaxation is mindfulness, which means paying attention to the present moment in a nonjudgmental manner.

- By mindfully directing your attention to your breathing, you can create mental relaxation, which is helpful with anxiety.

- When practicing mindfulness or PMR, be patient with yourself if you find this difficult. With practice, you'll get better at mastering these relaxation techniques!

Home Practice

- **PMR Practice:** Practice PMR at least *once per day* for at least *one week*. Track your progress in the following chart, monitoring your physical, mental, and overall relaxation. For now, your goal is to achieve at least a moderate amount of overall relaxation using this exercise, or around 50 on a 100-point scale.

- **Mindful Relaxation:** Practice mindful breathing or the mindful cloud exercise at least *once per day* for at least *one week*. Track your progress in the following chart. In addition to tracking your relaxation level during these exercises, take note of your degree of present-moment awareness, nonjudgment, and nonreactivity. Again, try to shoot for a moderate level (50 on a 100-point scale).

Progressive Muscle Relaxation Tracking

Rate your experience of progressive muscle relaxation in the chart below. Use a scale from 0 to 100, where 0 means not feeling relaxed at all and 100 means feeling completely relaxed. Moderate relaxation will be a 50 on this scale.

	Mon	Tue	Wed	Thu	Fri	Sat	Sun
Physical Relaxation (How much *less* body tension do you feel on a scale of 0–100?)							
Mental Relaxation (How mentally calm do you feel on a scale of 0–100?)							
Overall Relaxation (How much relaxation overall do you feel on a scale of 0–100?)							

Mindful Relaxation Tracking

Rate your experience of mindful breathing and the mindful cloud exercise in the chart below. Use a scale from 0 to 100, where 0 means not at all relaxed, not at all focused on the present, unable to let go of judgments, or unable to be nonreactive to thoughts, and 100 means completely relaxed, focused on the present, nonjudgmental, and nonreactive.

Mindful Breathing	Mon	Tue	Wed	Thu	Fri	Sat	Sun
Mental Relaxation (How mentally calm do you feel on a scale of 0–100?)							
Present Awareness (How much present-moment awareness do you feel on a scale of 0–100?)							
Nonjudgment (How much were you able to let go of judgments on a scale of 0–100?)							
Nonreactivity (How much were you able to not respond to your thoughts on a scale of 0–100?)							

Mindful Cloud Exercise	Mon	Tue	Wed	Thu	Fri	Sat	Sun
Mental Relaxation (How mentally calm do you feel on a scale of 0–100?)							
Present Awareness (How much present-moment awareness do you feel on a scale of 0–100?)							
Nonjudgment (How much were you able to let go of judgments on a scale of 0–100?)							
Nonreactivity (How much were you able to not respond to your thoughts on a scale of 0–100?)							

MODULE 3

Rethinking Thoughts

Imagine you are home alone. It's the end of a long day, and you are ready to relax. Your family members (or roommates) are away for the evening and not expected back anytime soon. You've just finished eating dinner and are sitting down to watch a movie. Suddenly you hear a door slam (adapted from Beck 1976). It goes on for a few seconds. *What goes through your mind in this exact moment?* What do you *automatically think* about the situation? Write what first popped into your mind in the space below:

Automatic thought: _____

Next, think about how you'd *feel* in this situation (scared, annoyed, excited) if that was your thought, and write it below:

Feeling: _____

Although your mind probably jumped to a particular thought right away when you read about the situation, there are numerous possible thoughts you could have had. In the space below, list some other interpretations of what could be happening. Then think about how you'd feel in response to that thought:

Thought: _____

Feeling: _____

Thought: _____

Feeling: _____

Thought: _____

Feeling: _____

If this was difficult, that's okay: sometimes coming up with different interpretations of a situation is hard. Some examples of different thoughts and their feelings could be:

- *Maybe one of my family members came home early,* which might make you feel *concerned*

- *Something might have broken and will need to be fixed,* which might leave you feeling *annoyed*

- *Maybe someone broke into the house,* which would likely cause *fear*

- *The wind blew the door shut,* which might leave you feeling *neutral* or *unconcerned*

As you can see, you could have several emotional responses to this situation depending on what you were thinking. This situation is inherently ambiguous, as are many situations in life. Thus, how you *feel* about a situation will depend on what you think and what conclusions you draw.

Anxious Thinking and the Anxiety Cycle

The idea that our thoughts and interpretations influence how we feel isn't new. In fact, Epictetus (55–135 CE), a Greek Stoic philosopher, was known to say: "People are not moved by things, but the view they take of them." Several centuries later, William Shakespeare said: "There is nothing either good or bad, but thinking makes it so." Recall in Section III of Module 1 ("How Anxiety Attacks") that we presented the three components of anxiety—physical, cognitive, and behavioral—and discussed how they affect each other and can create a vicious cycle of anxiety. Here we've begun to discuss this second aspect: the *cognitive* component of anxiety.

There are two important points we wish to make about this cycle. First, when people *think* in anxious ways, they're more likely to feel anxious and behave in anxious ways. Think back to Sofia, who worries about her children, and consider a situation in which she hasn't heard from her son in over a day. If she thinks, "I know he was at a party last night; what if he got hit by a drunk driver on his way home?" she's more likely to *feel* anxious and *behave* in anxious ways (repeatedly calling him, checking the police blotter from the night before).

Second, and as we also discussed in Section III of Module 1, when people experience chronic problematic anxiety and physical tension, they're more likely to *think* in anxious ways. Recall the example presented at the beginning of this section. If you were sitting down to watch a suspenseful horror movie and the lights were off, you'd probably be *more likely* to have an anxious thought about the strange noise than if you were watching a lighthearted comedy while it was still daylight outside. People with a high level of general anxiety react as if they're *always* watching a suspenseful movie. Because their body is in a constant state of tension and anxiety, they're more likely to produce anxious thoughts in response to ambiguous situations. This is because when the body is in a physically tense state, it's sending feedback to the brain that something is wrong. For example, Jill is more likely to assume that an ambiguous text from her friends means they're upset with her if she's already tense and anxious after a long, stressful day at work, whereas the same message might not bother her at all on a relaxing weekend morning. Does this mean her friends are *actually* more likely to be upset on a weeknight? Not at all. She's just more likely to *interpret* the ambiguous text in that way, which causes her anxiety.

Thus, it's not the situation but our *thoughts* (our interpretations of the situation) that drive our emotions and behaviors. A number of factors determine how we interpret things. Being chronically anxious and tense *increases the likelihood* of having anxious thoughts.

Automatic Thinking

Thoughts serve an important purpose—they help us evaluate situations, make quick judgments, form potential solutions, and consider what might happen if we acted a certain way. In fact, we're so dependent on thinking that sometimes we're hardly aware we're doing it! This is what we mean when we refer to *automatic thinking*.

Automatic thinking happens quickly and without conscious awareness. There is a reason for this: being able to think quickly is adaptive. You make hundreds of decisions in any given day, including what to eat, what to wear, how to get to work or school, what projects to work on at your job, what music to listen to, what to watch on TV, what time to go to bed...you get the idea. That's a lot of information for your brain to sort through! If the process of thinking were deliberate and slow, it would take us too long to assess a situation and determine our course of action. Much of the time, automatic thinking works very well for us. It's less effortful for our brain and lets us evaluate social situations, form quick judgments, and make efficient decisions.

However, sometimes automatic thinking creates unintended problems. Namely, our brain develops shortcuts that lead to errors and irrational conclusions. These mental shortcuts allow us to think efficiently, but they're prone to bias, and contribute to things like stereotypes and prejudice. Imagine you have to buy a birthday gift for your friend's five-year-old daughter and you assume she'd like a doll rather than a toy car. Although this may be a relatively benign example, stereotypes can sometimes be harmful because they're overgeneralized assumptions. In the same way, mental shortcuts can contribute to biases in thinking that lead to problematic anxiety.

Emotional Reasoning

Often, thoughts that "feel" threatening to us are more likely to be treated as "facts." For example, while Sofia is waiting for her son to return her call, she may feel so anxious that she assumes something terrible *must* have happened, even if there is no other evidence to suggest he's in danger. It's normal for threatening thoughts to be treated as accurate, hard-and-fast truths. In fact, our brains are hardwired to take threatening information seriously, because ignoring it could endanger our survival. Analyzing our way through situations based on *feelings* rather than *facts* is referred to as *emotional reasoning*.

Emotional reasoning is common for all people. Take automatic thinking—it's more efficient to think based on *emotion* than on *logic and reason* (which would require a much more substantial and effortful review of the information). Consider a person who has "a good feeling" about the lottery and purchases a scratch card, only to join millions of others in disappointment. Or another person who assumes her coworker is intentionally trying to "push her buttons" because she "had a feeling" that person didn't like her. Or a third person who "knows" his partner is cheating on him, simply because he "feels" jealous. All of these are examples of emotional reasoning, or assuming something is true simply because it feels true. When it comes to problematic anxiety, it's precisely *because* we're more likely to treat thoughts as facts when we're anxious that we need to examine our thoughts *when* we feel anxious.

Challenging Your Thoughts

The Roman emperor (and another Stoic philosopher) Markus Aurelius (121–180 CE), said: "If you are distressed by anything external, the pain isn't due to the thing itself, but to your estimate of it, and this you have the power to revoke at any moment." By "estimate," he means interpretation, which, as we discussed earlier, can influence the pain or anxious distress we experience. But Markus Aurelius took it a step further, by saying that we have the ability to reject the interpretations we make. This means we can do something about our thinking. We have the ability to slow down and become aware of automatic thoughts, and then evaluate whether they're actually realistic. Over the course of this module, we're going to teach you 1) how to identify problematic patterns of anxious thinking and 2) how to challenge your anxious thoughts. This will help you interrupt the vicious cycle of anxiety.

Because thinking is automatic and you've been thinking in the same way for a long time, these skills can be initially difficult to learn. Learning to observe your thinking is a skill that requires patience and practice. In the beginning, it will be hard to slow down and watch your thinking, but keep working at it. You're not alone! Remember, you can use your *feelings* of anxiety as a signal that there may be automatic, irrational, anxious thoughts under the surface that need to be examined. As you saw in the model of anxiety discussed in Section III of Module 1, thoughts about some possible bad outcome are a major component of feeling anxious, and often drive anxiety-related physical sensations and behaviors. So, even if you're not aware of exactly what the thoughts are, use your feelings as an indicator that it's time to slow down and pay attention to your thoughts. If you do this consistently, you'll start to notice more patterns and the thoughts will become easier to detect.

Anxious Thinking Traps

All people (even people without problematic anxiety) are prone to fall into thinking "traps." These thinking traps are inevitable because we use thinking shortcuts, and most of the time these shortcuts don't cause any problems for us. However, sometimes these shortcuts create difficulties like problematic and unrelenting anxiety. For people with problematic anxiety there are two primary thinking traps: *probability overestimation* and *catastrophizing*. We'll explore both of these in more detail.

Probability Overestimation

Probability overestimation is one of the most common types of thinking traps for people with problematic anxiety. Probability overestimation involves making an inaccurate or unreasonable prediction that an unlikely event is highly probable. People who fall into this trap confuse *possibility* with *probability*. A common example of probability overestimation is the fear of getting on an airplane because the plane might fatally crash. For people who experience this type of fear, the likelihood of a crash may feel quite high. However, air travel is one of the safest modes of transportation. In the last ten years, there have been approximately 300 plane crashes on commercial passenger flights. This may seem high, but there are an estimated 100,000 flights *per day*, or 3.5 million flights *per year*. Thus, the probability of a plane crash over the past ten years was roughly 0.0000004, or less than one in a million (Aviation Safety 2018). If you consider that less than a third of airplane accidents result in fatalities, the probability of a fatal plane crash decreases further. You can see where this is going: although an airplane crash is *possible*, it's extremely unlikely.

Let's consider another example from one of your workbook companions, Sofia:

Sofia is at home writing an email to a friend. Suddenly, she feels a sharp pain on the back of her head. The pain is intermittently sharp and throbbing. She begins to get tense in her shoulders and starts rubbing her neck and head. Her mouth gets dry. She's thinking to herself, "What if I'm having a stroke?" She closes the email and begins to do an Internet search of her symptoms. She calls her husband to see if he thinks she should take herself to the doctor or call 911. She begins to get panicky.

You should be able to recognize each component of the anxiety cycle. Sofia is experiencing anxious thoughts ("What if I'm having a stroke?"), anxious physical sensations (tension, dry mouth), and anxious behaviors (researching her symptoms, calling her husband). Importantly, Sofia is feeling anxious and behaving in anxious ways *precisely* because she's interpreting ambiguous physical sensations (throbbing) as life threatening. If Sofia were to think to herself, "I must be getting a headache," she'd probably take some medicine and resume her activities without any worry. Remember, anxious thinking leads to anxious feelings and behaviors. Sofia is feeling panicky because she *believes* she might be having a stroke. Sofia is falling into the common thinking trap of *probability overestimation,* assuming that an unlikely event (having a stroke) is highly probable. Sofia is also engaging in emotional reasoning: she *feels* anxious about the pain and so she believes it *must be true* that something is wrong. Anxious feelings have led her brain to come up with an anxiety-based conclusion. Luckily, we can help Sofia adjust her thinking and interrupt this vicious anxiety cycle. Let's take a look at how this works.

Challenging Probability Overestimation

To counter probability overestimation, you'll need to learn to consider other facts and possibilities about an anxiety-inducing situation *without* jumping to conclusions or making overly broad generalizations. Sofia has jumped to a conclusion ("I'm having a stroke") without considering all of the facts and possibilities. Considering other possibilities and evaluating the evidence is crucial because judgments and predictions based on emotional reasoning are very likely to be biased.

There are five steps to counter probability overestimation. We'll walk through each step, using Sofia's fear of a stroke as an example to illustrate how this works in practice.

Step 1. Observe your thinking and treat thoughts as *hypotheses*. The first step to changing anything is becoming aware that it's happening. This is certainly true with our thinking, because as we pointed out earlier, it happens automatically, quickly, and often outside of our immediate awareness. Use your anxious feelings as an indicator that there are anxious thoughts lurking beneath the surface.

Once you've observed that you are feeling anxious, write down your thoughts on the Challenging Probability Overestimation worksheet provided at the end of this section and at http://www.newharbinger.com/44529. Writing will help you get better at *slowing down* and *observing* your thoughts. When you write a thought down, ask yourself, "How believable is this thought?" We suggest you rate the initial believability of the thought on a scale of 0 (not at all believable) to 100 (completely believable, absolutely true). In the beginning, especially in more anxious moments, it's likely that you'll rate your thoughts as relatively highly believable, in the 75 to 100 range. This is normal. Remember, our brains are hardwired to treat thoughts as facts. If you have difficulty identifying your anxious thoughts, remember that they usually come in the form of predictions about something going wrong in the future ("If…happens, then…"). Review "The Cognitive Component of Anxiety" if you need further review about identifying your thoughts.

Let's take a look at Sofia's example, which might look something like this:

Situation	Thought (How believable is the thought from 0–100?)	Physical Sensations & Feelings	Behavior	SUDS
Head begins throbbing	I'm having a stroke (80)	Dry mouth, tension, panic	Researching symptoms, call husband	85

You'll see we also included space to note physical sensations and behaviors. Even though we're focusing on thoughts in this module, identifying physical sensations is good practice for better understanding your anxiety cycle, and can also help you detect emotional reasoning.

Step 2. Evaluate the evidence *for* and the evidence *against* the prediction. Now begin to evaluate the evidence that supports or refutes your thinking. This will help you think in more rational, rather than emotional, ways. What is evidence, exactly? Evidence is fact-driven. It's based on objective information you could present to a judge in court, rather than "feelings" or opinions. When we're highly anxious, it's easy to engage in *emotional reasoning,* which causes us to treat subjective feelings as evidence. But evidence is observable or verifiable to others, meaning that it's not based on our perspective alone. When examining evidence, avoid subjective thoughts and feelings, and stick to the facts! Let's return to Sofia's example. Which of the following might be evidence to support Sofia's thought?

☐ Family history of vascular disease

☐ Head pain

☐ "I think my vision became blurry"

☐ "I've never felt pain quite like this before"

The first two would be examples of evidence because they're observable, verifiable, and based on facts rather than perceptions. The second two are interpretations, and thus don't count as evidence. Sofia's thought about never feeling pain like this before is based on a subjective perception, likely biased by her fear about what this pain means. She can't objectively compare her current pain to past experiences, so it's not good evidence. All she can say is that she has head pain.

Finding evidence "against" a particular thought can be more challenging because it requires considering alternative ideas that are not as natural or automatic. All human beings are prone to seek information that supports their beliefs and ignore, or discount, information that goes against them, a phenomenon called *confirmation bias.* This is especially difficult when we're experiencing problematic anxiety. Stay with it though, and be patient with yourself, especially in the beginning. You can also get the perspective of someone else to help you generate evidence, as an outside perspective can look for more objective evidence. Can you think of possible evidence that would go against Sofia's thought that she's having a stroke? Let's take a look at Sofia's chart for evidence for and against:

Evidence For	Evidence Against
Family history of stroke	Relatively young
Head pain	Healthy lifestyle
	No other symptoms of stroke

Step 3. Explore alternative possibilities and evaluate their evidence. Now it's time to consider alternative possibilities or explanations. Again, we want to emphasize that this is a difficult skill that doesn't come naturally to most people. Most of us are not used to thinking in a deliberate and rational manner when feeling anxious. However, this is the most important time to use this skill, because this is when you are most likely to think in biased ways! Consider some of these questions to help you formulate alternative possibilities:

- What explanation(s) would I suggest to a friend?

- What led me to believe this, and are there other conclusions?

- What might be another explanation for [head pain]?

- What else might cause [head pain]?

- If someone else were experiencing [head pain], what would I think?

Before checking back in with Sofia, can you think of some possible *alternative* explanations for her head pain? Continue reading below to see what she came up with.

Alternatives	Evidence For	Evidence Against
It's the start of a headache My eyes are strained from staring at the computer I'm fatigued It's nothing	Head pain Prone to headaches Have been on the computer for a long time Didn't sleep enough last night Sometimes bodies do random things	Eyes don't feel dry and tired Don't feel tired Head pain

This step is perhaps the most difficult part of the exercise. It's common for people to feel like this part is *forced* or *phony*. Having worked with many people with problematic anxiety, we often hear people say, "Well, yes, but it doesn't feel true" or "It's not genuine" or "I still don't believe it." This isn't a reason to give up on the exercise. In fact, it's a sign that you are doing it correctly. This is because you are actually thinking about other possible explanations rather than just reacting to your initial automatic thought. If all of the alternative explanations "felt" true, you wouldn't be anxious and likely wouldn't have needed to go through the exercise to begin with. Human beings engage in emotional reasoning out of habit and so it will take time to get skilled at this exercise. Stay with it!

Step 4. Determine the real probability. Now you can determine or calculate the *real probability*. Using available information, you'll determine the actual likelihood of the predicted, negative outcome. This is done by assessing how many times the event has actually occurred divided by the number of times you've found yourself in a similar situation or have had a similar worry about the feared outcome. You might ask yourself, "How many times has X happened or not happened?" In this case, Sofia would determine the number of times she's had a stroke (0 times) and divide that by the number of times she's experienced head pain. Calculating this second portion can involve some estimating, but it's an important part of this exercise, so don't give up too quickly. Let's work through Sofia's example together. Sofia estimates that she has 2 headaches per month (or 24 headaches per year). She doesn't remember having had headaches as a young woman, but she's experienced regular headaches and pains since her mid-twenties. Therefore, she estimates 24 headaches per year, multiplied by 30 years, which is a total of 720 headaches in her adult life. Thus, the real probability is 0 out of 720. Determining the real probability will provide actual data (rather than emotional data) to inform your thinking. Take a look at Sofia's form:

A.	How many times has this situation occurred [head pain] or how many times have I had this thought?	720
B.	How many times has it come true? How many times has [feared outcome] happened?	0
C.	What is the real probability? (Divide the number in "B" by the number in "A.")	0%

Step 5. Generate an alternative, more likely interpretation. The final step is to generate an alternative, more realistic thought. Start by reviewing the information you gathered in steps 2 through 4. What do you make of the evidence, the alternative explanations, and the real probability? Ask yourself the following question: "What is a more realistic possibility?" What alternative interpretations can you generate for Sofia? Finish the exercise by rating the believability of the new thoughts on a scale from 0 (not at all believable) to 100 (completely believable, absolutely true). We also suggest you go back and *re*-rate the believability of the initial thought you had. Let's take a look at the final part of Sofia's form:

	Thoughts	Believability
After reviewing the evidence, rate the believability of the original thought.	Original Thought: I'm having a stroke .	35
What is a more realistic possibility? Rate the believability of this thought.	Alternative Thought: It seems much more likely that I'm just fatigued or getting a headache.	60
What can I tell myself in the future?	While it's certainly possible that something could be wrong, the evidence suggests that's pretty unlikely.	60

Additional Considerations

We wish to emphasize three important points about generating alternative thoughts. At first, it's not uncommon for people to *feel* like the alternative thoughts, which they generate at the end of the exercise, are not fully believable. This is because of the nature of emotional reasoning. It's simply easier for our brains to *think* in anxious ways when we're *feeling* anxious. Remember, our brains are hardwired to take anxious feelings seriously and so it's difficult for our brains to think in alternative (or non-anxious) ways when we feel anxious. Nonetheless, check and see if doing this exercise changes the believability of your original anxious thought at all. Even small changes are major progress! With repeated practice and consideration of the alternatives, the believability will continue to decrease.

The second point worth emphasizing is that countering anxious thoughts is *not* the same as "positive thinking" or replacing "bad" thoughts with "good" ones. In fact, the purpose of this exercise is *not* to generate biased thoughts in the other direction. For example, we wouldn't encourage Sofia to arrive at the conclusion "I'm perfectly fine and nothing bad will ever happen to me!" This would be unreasonable and truly artificial, because it's not based on evidence either. Instead, the goal is to look at the evidence for and against an automatic thought, and then come up with a more *realistic* alternative.

Finally, when going through the steps for challenging probability overestimation, you may find that steps 2, 3, and 4 are more or less useful, or even become redundant, for certain thoughts. For example, calculating the actual odds of a plane crash might be particularly helpful, whereas evaluating evidence for alternative explanations might do the trick when you hear a noise above you when you are home alone. If that happens, then do what works best for you. The important thing is that you are 1) questioning your automatic thoughts, and 2) considering possible alternatives.

In conclusion, probability overestimation involves making an inaccurate or unreasonable prediction that an unlikely event is highly probable. Probability overestimation can be countered by evaluating the evidence *for* and *against* the thought, exploring alternative explanations, and calculating the real probability.

Section Review: Key Points

- Thoughts, rather than situations alone, drive our emotions and behaviors. Being chronically anxious and tense increases the likelihood of having anxious thoughts.

- Automatic thoughts are thoughts that occur quickly and often without conscious awareness. These thoughts can easily be biased, such as when we're making judgments about situations based on *feelings* rather than *facts*. This is called emotional reasoning.

- Thinking traps are common, even for people without high levels of anxiety. One of the most common thinking traps for people with anxiety is probability overestimation, which involves exaggerating the likelihood that a bad outcome will happen.

- Individuals can counter probability overestimation by considering the evidence for and against an anxious thought, estimating the actual odds that a negative outcome will occur, and generating alternative explanations and more probable possibilities.

Home Practice

- **Challenge Probability Overestimation:** Continue self-monitoring, but this week use the Challenging Probability Overestimation form on the next page to practice challenging your thoughts. Try to fill out the form for at least three probability overestimation thoughts.

Challenging Probability Overestimation

STEP 1: Observe your thinking.

Situation	Thought (How believable is the thought from 0–100?)	Physical Sensations & Feelings	Behavior	SUDS

STEP 2: Evaluate the evidence "for" and "against" the thought in Column 2.

Evidence For	Evidence Against

STEP 3: Explore alternative possibilities and evaluate their evidence.

Alternatives	Evidence For	Evidence Against

STEP 4: Determine the real probability.

A.	How many times has this situation occurred or how many times have I had this thought?	
B.	How many times has it come true? How many times has [feared outcome] happened?	
C.	What is the real probability? (Divide the number in "B" by the number in "A.")	

STEP 5: Generate an alternative interpretation and re-rate the believability of the initial thought.

	Thoughts	Believability
After reviewing the evidence, rate the believability of the original thought.	Original Thought:	
What is a more realistic possibility? Rate the believability of this thought.	Alternative Thought:	
What can I tell myself in the future?		

Catastrophizing

Sometimes people find that even when they've accurately assessed the likelihood of a something going wrong, they're still anxious because the negative outcome they're worrying about feels unbearable. This leads us to a second common thinking trap that affects anxious individuals, which we call *catastrophizing* or *catastrophic thinking*. Catastrophic thinking involves two errors in thinking: 1) assuming an undesirable situation is intolerable and 2) underestimating your ability to cope. Essentially, catastrophic thinking is making a big deal out of something that's not a big deal. Because of the effect of emotional reasoning, it's common for individuals who are feeling anxious to assume a bad situation is a disaster. However, true catastrophes are situations that can't be rectified, and they're extremely rare. Losing a loved one in an accident suddenly is a catastrophe. Being unable to feed yourself and your children is a catastrophe. But forgetting to pay the bills isn't a catastrophe. Being late to an appointment isn't a catastrophe. Even losing a job isn't necessarily a catastrophe. It's a bad situation, but it can be rectified.

Adopting a thinking style that turns everything into a crisis, even if it isn't, is called catastrophic thinking. Consider thinking of bad situations on a spectrum ranging from mild inconveniences to true catastrophes. We offer a "Spectrum of Catastrophes" below, which shows where certain negative events are likely to fall for most people with regard to the true severity of the outcome, and the intensity of the emotion justified. Obviously, the exact placement of the events on this scale is somewhat subjective and will vary based on your personal circumstances and values, so consider creating your own "Spectrum of Catastrophes" with personalized anchor points along the scale.

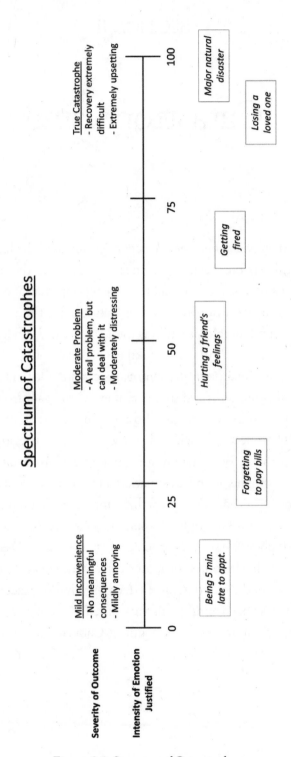

Figure 3.1. *Spectrum of Catastrophes*

Let's take a look at an example from your workbook companion, Jill:

It's a Friday afternoon and Jill is preparing to go home for the weekend. She's been looking forward to meeting up with friends for dinner and going to an exercise class on Sunday. At five o'clock, she receives an email from her boss requesting a report for a client by Monday. The boss explains that this report can be a rough draft, but it's necessary to have by Monday morning because this client has VIP status. Jill's face gets warm, her chest tightens, and her breathing gets shallow. She immediately begins thinking that this is awful. She thinks there is no way she will be able to turn in a good report in time and assumes that the report, whatever she's able to get done, will be of terrible quality. She decides to cancel all of her plans immediately and stays at work until 10 p.m. with plans to return the next morning. Throughout the evening, while she works, she finds herself having intrusive and uncontrollable worries that the report will be an incomplete and poorly written product. She's also worrying about how this job is affecting her quality of life and ability to sleep. She feels the entire situation is unbearable and as a result she feels anxious, irritable, and stressed.

Can you recognize each component of the anxiety cycle? Jill is experiencing anxious thoughts and worries about her ability to produce a quality report on time as well as the impact it has on her life. She's experiencing physical sensations of anxiety (flushing face, tight chest muscles, shortness of breath) and anxious behaviors (canceling all social plans, staying late). Importantly, Jill is feeling anxious and behaving in anxious ways *precisely* because she's interpreting the potential negative outcome in this situation (turning in a subpar report) as a disaster. Because she believes a less-than-perfect report would be unacceptable, she works late and cancels her plans, which further exacerbates her anxiety about the job. Her anxious thinking leads to anxious feelings and behaviors, which in turn makes the worries even stronger, and she begins thinking that the situation is intolerable. Jill is falling into the common thinking trap of *catastrophizing*. Jill is assuming that turning in an unfinished product will be a crisis, even though her boss indicated this would be okay. Luckily, we can help Jill correct this destructive thinking pattern and interrupt this vicious anxiety cycle. Let's take a look at how this works.

Challenging Catastrophic Thinking

To challenge catastrophic thinking, it's necessary to slow the mind down and consider the *actual severity* of an outcome as well as what you'd realistically do to cope *if* the situation were to come true. Remember, it's important to remember that anxious, catastrophic thinking is highly likely to be biased because, like *probability overestimation*, it's based on emotional reasoning. We're going to introduce a specific method to challenge catastrophic thinking called the "so what" approach, which involves thinking through the actual consequences of the feared outcome occurring in order to determine its actual severity and identify ways to cope. There are three specific steps to countering catastrophic thinking. Let's return to Jill's situation to demonstrate how this works in practice.

Step 1. Observe your thinking and treat thoughts as *hypotheses*. Remember, awareness is the first step to behavior change. To challenge catastrophic thinking, you must first be aware that it's happening. Just like *probability overestimation*, *catastrophizing* happens quickly in the form of an automatic thought. Remember, your anxious feelings are a good indicator of possibly biased, anxious thoughts. Once you've observed that you are feeling anxious, write down your thoughts on paper. For catastrophic thinking, we suggest you use the Challenging Catastrophic Thinking worksheet provided at the end of this module and at http://www.newharbinger.com/44529. We encourage you to hand write your thoughts to facilitate slowing down and increasing awareness. As you write each thought, ask yourself, "How believable is this thought?" and then rate the initial believability of the thought on a scale of 0 (not at all believable) to 100 (completely believable, absolutely true).

Let's take a look at Jill's example, which might look something like this:

Situation	Thought (How believable is the thought from 0–100?)	Physical Sensations & Feelings	Behavior	SUDS
Boss asks for report on Friday afternoon	This report will be completely terrible (100)	Face flushed, tension, shortness of breath	Cancel plans, work late	95

Step 2. Determine the actual severity of the outcome. Now identify the true severity of the feared outcome. When people engage in catastrophic thinking, they tend to exaggerate the severity. To assist you in realistically appraising the severity of the situation, try asking yourself

"so what?" The "so what" approach shouldn't be confused with a "who cares?" attitude. We're not suggesting that you shouldn't care about whether bad things happen or not. Rather, the goal is to develop a realistic perspective on the actual consequences of a negative outcome. Think of the "so what" approach as a method of asking questions like, "So what happens next?" and "If that happens, then what?" This approach is about following the thought through to its logical outcome and then asking yourself, "So how bad would that be, really?" We return to Jill to see how this works:

Questions to Ask Yourself	Your Responses
What are you afraid will happen?	The report won't be finished in time and I'll give my boss a terrible product.
And, so what will happen next, if that occurs?	My boss could be upset with me.
If that happens, what will come next?	My boss would probably talk to me, might ask what's wrong.
Would anything else happen?	The client might be disappointed, could choose to leave? Boss could be more upset.

Step 3. Identify your coping strategies. Now identify your coping strategies—that is, what you could do if the outcome were to come true. This is a crucial step because individuals who catastrophize typically forget about the resources they have to deal with a situation if it were to happen. You are less likely to think something is a big deal if you feel confident in your ability to handle it! To guide you in identifying your coping skills and strategies, there are several questions you can ask yourself. Consider these questions for Jill, who is catastrophizing her work situation:

Questions to Ask Yourself	Your Responses
Has this [feared outcome] ever happened before?	One time I turned in a report that was missing a section and I didn't even realize it. Have never lost a client before.
What did you do before?	Apologized and then completed the missing section ; boss was not even upset.
What could you do if this happened?	I could talk with my boss about how to improve it. We could make sure we have enough time to do a better job next time. Couldn't do much if we lost the client.
Who could you rely on to help you get through it if it were to occur?	My boss (we have a good relationship and would get through it), coworkers, friends.
What skills or resources could you apply if that happened?	Hardworking, open to feedback, would try to address it with boss.

Step 4. Generate an alternative, more likely interpretation. Just as we did in the previous section, the final step is to generate an alternative, more realistic thought. To do this, consider your responses to the "so what" exercise. Review your coping strategies. What do you make of the evidence you've collected? To guide you through this step, ask yourself the following questions: "How severe is the situation, actually?" "What is your ability to cope?" "What can you tell yourself in the future?" Finish this exercise by rating the believability of these alternative statements. What do you think of Jill's situation? Let's take a look at her responses below:

	Alternative Thoughts	Believability
How severe is the situation, actually, on a scale of 0–100?	It wouldn't feel good to turn in an incomplete report, but there wasn't much time, so it's not an actual reflection of my skills (20/100).	90
	Losing a client wouldn't be great, but the firm would be just fine (40/100).	90
	I wouldn't like it if my boss was upset at me but we'd recover (30/100).	75
What do you make of your ability to cope?	I would get through it because my boss and I have a good relationship and I have supportive friends.	80
What can you tell yourself in the future?	I don't do my best work under this pressure, but it's not a crisis if I don't turn in a perfect product.	80

Additional Considerations

We should emphasize a final important point about catastrophic thinking. It's difficult to consider all of your coping abilities, especially when feeling anxious.. To assist you, we've listed below some examples of coping skills and strategies, resources, and personal characteristics that you should remind yourself of if you find yourself engaging in catastrophic thinking. You'll notice that some of the items on this list will apply in some situations but not others. Read this list and circle any that apply to you.

- Resilience
- Strong social support network
- Ability to solve problems
- Supportive coworkers
- Sense of humor
- Dependability
- Determination
- Intelligence
- Ambition
- Good social skills
- Organized
- Good at delegating
- Cooperative
- Honest
- Stable living situation
- Supportive spouse or partner
- Creativity
- Physical health
- Close family relationships
- Highly specialized or unique skill set
- Religious beliefs
- Trustworthy
- Interpersonal warmth
- Access to health care
- Hardworking
- Detail oriented
- Understanding boss
- Team player
- Willingness to learn
- Open to feedback
- Education
- Multiple, varied hobbies and interests
- Optimistic
- Flexibility
- Able to multitask
- Good time-management skills
- Good listener
- Motivated
- Versatile skills
- Persevering
- Open-minded
- Integrity

Can you think of others you could add to this list? Commit to revisiting this list the next time you are thinking in catastrophic ways.

Combining Probability Overestimation and Catastrophizing

Often both probability overestimation and catastrophic thinking are present in our anxious thoughts. This is because people assume a negative outcome is much more like than it actually is, *and then* assume the outcome would result in disaster if it came true. Consider an example from Elijah, who worries about his graduate schoolwork: *I'll miss the deadline for the assignment and get a poor grade in the class* or *I'll stumble over my words during the presentation and blush.* In such situations it can be helpful to break the thought into two separate thoughts and use the techniques described above for each individual part. For example, *I'll miss the deadline* and *I'll stumble over my words* are instances of probability overestimation. You could target these by examining the evidence for and against such beliefs, and calculate the odds that these things will happen, because the probability of them occurring may not be as high as you initially think. Let's take a look at how this would work for Elijah using the first thought, "I'll miss the deadline for the assignment and get a poor grade."

In Step 1, he'd begin to observe his thought and identify the various components of his worry. Here, he also labels each component of the thought to guide him through the exercise.

Situation	Thought (How believable is the thought from 0–100?)	Physical Sensations & Feelings	Behavior	SUDS
Starting a school assignment	I'll miss the deadline (probability overestimation) and get a poor grade (catastrophizing) (75)	Chest tightness, shortness of breath, neck pain, anxiety	Procrastinate, play video games	70

In Step 2, he'd begin to observe his thought and identify the various components of his worry. Can you think of other things Elijah could include?

Evidence for thought "I'll miss the deadline"	Evidence against thought "I'll miss the deadline"
I have a limited amount of time before the deadline.	I have only missed one assignment in years of school.
I have many other commitments and assignments.	I still have time before the deadline.

In Step 3, Elijah begins to consider alternative explanations and examines the evidence for and against these alternatives. Read on to see what he came up with. Test yourself—can you think of some alternatives for Elijah?

Alternatives	Evidence For	Evidence Against
I won't miss the deadline, but it won't be very good work.	I have never missed a deadline before in this class.	I'm running out of time.
I'll get the assignment done, I won't miss the deadline, and it will be just fine.	I have done good work in this class before.	I have never experienced an emergency that stopped me from getting work done.
I'll turn the assignment in late.	I'm running out of time.	
An emergency will come up and I won't be able to complete the assignment and will miss the deadline.		

The fourth step is to determine or calculate the *real probability* to provide actual data (rather than emotional data) to inform your thinking. In this case, the likelihood of missing the deadline is determined by looking at how many assignments Elijah has had and determining how many times he's actually missed the deadline. He estimates the situation based on how many classes he's taken in his school program so far (20) and how many deadlines he's had per class (he estimates 3). Here is what Elijah wrote down for his prediction that he will miss the deadline:

A.	How many times has this situation occurred [class assignment] or how many times have I had this thought?	60
B.	How many times has it come true? How many times has [feared outcome] happened?	2
C.	What is the real probability? (Divide the number in "B" by the number in "A.")	3%

In the final step Elijah arrives at an alternative, more realistic thought. What is a more realistic possibility for Elijah?

	Thoughts	**Believability**
After reviewing the evidence, rate the believability of the original thought.	Original Thought: *I'm going to miss the deadline.*	15
What is a more realistic possibility? Rate the believability of this thought.	Alternative Thought: *It seems much more likely that I'll turn something in by the deadline.*	75
What can I tell myself in the future?	*It's unlikely that I'll miss the deadline; this has rarely happened in the past.*	80

Then, you could work on de-catastrophizing the feared outcome, in this case, Elijah's fear of *getting a poor grade*. We return to Elijah's initial automatic thought, focusing on the component of the thought that involves catastrophizing:

Situation	Thought (How believable is the thought from 0–100?)	Physical Sensations & Feelings	Behavior	SUDS
Working on class assignment	I'll get a poor grade (100)	Chest tightness, shortness of breath, neck pain, anxiety	Procrastinate, play video games	70

Can you help Elijah evaluate the actual severity of this possible outcome?

Questions to Ask Yourself	Your Responses
What are you afraid will happen?	I'll get a poor grade.
And, so what will happen next, if that occurs?	My professor will be disappointed.
If that happens, what will come next?	I might fail the class.
Would anything else happen?	I could lose my scholarship.

After going through this exercise, Elijah determines that on the "Spectrum of Catastrophes," this is a 50 because it would be very disappointing, but not a crisis.

Next, Elijah generates a list of coping strategies he could use if his feared outcome were to come true.

Questions to Ask Yourself	Your Responses
Has this [feared outcome] ever happened before?	I've gotten below-average grades before, but I've never failed a class.
What did you do before?	Made up the work with extra credit.
What could you do if this happened?	I could talk to my professor about improving my grade. If I lost my scholarship, I could search for other funding support or ask my parents for help.
Who could you rely on to help you get through it if it were to occur?	My professor would help me. Friends and parents would also assist if asked.
What skills or resources could you apply if that happened?	Resourceful, good at problem solving; could get another roommate to reduce living expenses (if lost scholarship).

In the final step, Elijah reviews what he considered in the previous steps and comes up with some alternative, more realistic thoughts:

	Alternative Thoughts	Believability
How severe is the situation, actually, on a scale of 0–100?	It would be disappointing to get a poor grade and in the worst-case scenario I would fail the class. This would be disappointing, but not a crisis. I would work on other ways to improve my grade and situation and I have a lot of people who could help me.	75 90
What do you make of your ability to cope?	I'm resourceful and motivated to problem solve; I can deal with whatever happens.	80
What can you tell yourself in the future?	Even if I get a poor grade, it's not the end of the world.	80

Putting it all together, Elijah now has several more realistic ways of looking at the situation. Mainly, missing the deadline completely seems unlikely, and even if it happens, it won't be a crisis.

In some cases, a thought could be both overestimating a probability and catastrophizing at the *same time*. In this case, getting a poor grade was a catastrophic way of thinking, but may have also been probability overestimation. For instance, how likely are you to get a poor grade if you miss one deadline? It's okay to test an automatic thought's believability by going through the steps for both probability overestimation *and* catastrophizing. Both will help you come up with more reasonable and helpful alternative thoughts to tell yourself in anxious situations.

In a related way, you might also be asking at this point, "What if I can't tell the difference between *probability overestimation* and *catastrophizing?*" First, it's more important that you begin to learn to slow down and notice and challenge your thinking than it is to precisely categorize each thought perfectly accurately. Furthermore, you'll find that the techniques we've provided for challenging your thinking often work sufficiently well for problematic anxious thoughts of all types. What is most important is that you recognize your anxious thought patterns, and then challenge those thoughts to identify a more realistic or helpful alternative viewpoint.

Section Review: Key Points

- Catastrophizing involves assuming a situation is intolerable and underestimating your ability to cope.

- You can counter catastrophizing by evaluating the actual severity of the feared outcome and identifying coping strategies if the outcome were to come true. Remember that true catastrophes are rare, and involve situations that are extremely difficult to rectify.

- Challenging your catastrophic thinking allows you to see that even if a feared outcome occurs, it may not be as devastating as you initially thought.

- Anxious thoughts can include elements of both probability overestimation *and* catastrophizing. In these cases, it can be helpful to break a thought up into two individual thoughts.

- If you consider both types of common thinking traps and objectively challenge them, worry thoughts will often turn out to be less worrisome after all. The same skills can be applied to all types of anxious thinking traps.

Home Practice

- **Challenge Catastrophic Thinking:** Continue self-monitoring, but this week use the Challenging Catastrophic Thinking form on the next-page. Practice challenging at least three catastrophic thoughts. If thoughts arise in which both catastrophizing and probability overestimation are present, you can try using the probability overestimation exercise from the previous section as well.

Challenging Catastrophic Thinking

STEP 1: Observe your thinking.

Situation	Thought (How believable is the thought from 0–100?)	Physical Sensations & Feelings	Behavior	SUDS

STEP 2: Determine the actual severity of the outcome.

Questions to Ask Yourself	Your Responses
What are you afraid will happen?	
And, so what will happen next, if that occurs?	
If that happens, what will come next?	
Would anything else happen?	

STEP 3: Identify coping strategies.

Questions to Ask Yourself	Your Responses
Has this [feared outcome] ever happened before?	
What did you do before?	
What might you do if this happened?	
Who could you rely on to help you get through it if it were to occur?	
What skills or resources could you apply if that happened?	

STEP 4: Generate an alternative interpretation and re-rate the believability of the initial thought.

	Alternative Thoughts	Believability
How severe is the situation, actually, on a scale of 0–100?		
What do you make of your ability to cope?		
What can you tell yourself in the future?		

MODULE 4

Worries About Worries

Jill is about to meet two of her best friends for dinner for some long overdue catch-up time. She's been looking forward to this dinner for some time, but just as she arrives at the restaurant, a thought pops into her head about the presentation she has to give at work at the end of the week: "I'm not prepared yet, and the presentation is in two days! If I really want this presentation to go well, I should be working on this right now!" Her anxiety immediately increases, but she remembers her cognitive reappraisal skills. She realizes she's overestimating the probability that she won't have enough time to finish preparing tomorrow, and reminds herself that when she's done these presentations before, they've gone well. This helps some, but the thought that she should be preparing keeps popping back into her head. She remembers that for the last presentation she was extremely worried about not being prepared, so she spent the whole week getting ready. As a result, Jill wonders if she should be even more worried than she is. She thinks, "In the past, my worries helped me prepare for these presentations, because they seem to go well when I worry about them." She tries to just push these thoughts away, but they keep coming back and she finds that rather than enjoying her time with her friends, she keeps getting distracted by her anxiety. This frustrates her and makes her feel like she's not being a good friend (one of her other worries), so she stays until her friends want to go home. Her worry continues to bother her, however, and she heads home feeling disappointed that once again, anxiety got in the way of having a good time.

Detached Awareness

In the previous module, you learned how to challenge the thoughts that drive your anxiety by asking yourself questions about 1) the actual likelihood of the bad outcome you were worrying about (targeting *probability overestimation*) and 2) your ability to cope with that outcome if it did occur (targeting *catastrophizing*). This is a really powerful tool, but sometimes there are other thoughts or beliefs that get in the way of effectively challenging your anxious thoughts.

Beliefs About Thoughts

This week, we're going to start evaluating your *metacognitions,* which are your beliefs about your thoughts and worries. Learning to evaluate your metacognitions is similar to the process of cognitive restructuring because it involves examining the way you think. However, rather than focusing on whether the content of your thought is accurate, we're going to focus on your *relationship to your worries* and whether your *beliefs about your worries and thoughts* are helpful. For example, earlier we looked at the true odds and realistic outcomes of your worries (How likely is it that you'll actually fail the exam? Even if you did fail, how bad of an outcome would that actually be? What resources would help you cope?). In this section, we're not going to challenge the content of these worries. Instead, we're going to challenge your beliefs that you *should* be worried about these things. These beliefs are important because they can cause you to focus all your attention on your anxiety-producing automatic thoughts. Effectively addressing these beliefs can help you move past that anxiety and focus on living the life you want.

To make this clearer, let's go back to Jill. At dinner, whenever the thought about her work project popped into her head, it sent a surge of anxiety through her body that signaled, "Watch out, your presentation might go really poorly because you haven't prepared enough!" To Jill, that thought felt very important because she was reminded of the time when her anxiety drove her to prepare all week, and things ended up going well. As a result, she felt like she should listen to her anxiety. She believed her worry was helpful. It was hard for Jill to dismiss the "worry" thought, even when she realized that it was not all that realistic.

In this example, Jill had a *belief about her anxious thought*, or a *metacognition*. She thought that paying attention to her anxious thought was necessary to help her prepare for the perceived danger of possibly doing poorly on her presentation. Metacognitions are important because, just like they did for Jill, they can feed the worry cycle and make it very difficult to put the brakes on. Let's break it down more specifically, by considering the following thought of Jill's:

*"Last time I was super worried about the presentation,
so I spent the entire week preparing. That's why I did well."*

Jill is attributing her success to her worry-driven behavior, and therefore has developed a belief about the positive value of worry. This is what we call a positive metacognition, which is a belief that worry is helpful or beneficial. You can imagine how such beliefs might make it harder to let go of worry. Jill wouldn't want to completely let her worry go if she thinks it's doing something useful for her.

Below are some other examples of positive metacognitions. Identify and check examples that feel true for you. Be sure to write in any additional ways that you feel anxiety or worry is beneficial for you.

Positive Beliefs About Worry

☐ Worry helps prepare me for bad outcomes.

☐ Worry makes me feel in control.

☐ If I'm not worrying about a bad outcome, I'll be blindsided when it happens.

☐ Worry shows that I care.

☐ Worrying helps me avoid future problems.

☐ Worrying helps me perform better.

☐ Worry ensures I won't forget about something important.

☐ Other: _____

☐ Other: _____

Now you may better understand why it's been so difficult for you to stop worrying! Many people who worry a lot have these sorts of beliefs without even realizing it. Even though worry isn't fun, it can *feel* helpful in some way. Or at the very least, the idea of not worrying about possible bad things happening can feel even scarier than worry itself. Like the old saying goes, better the devil you know than the one you don't, right?

Well let's take a closer look at this. Although these positive beliefs about worry are understandable, to effectively reduce your anxiety it's important to see whether such beliefs really add up. To start, let's think about the *costs* of worry to see how they stack up against the perceived benefits. Below, take a few moments to list all the negative consequences that worry has on your life (on your energy levels, relationships, productivity).

Costs of Worry

- _____

- _____

- _____

- _____

- _____

- _____

- _____

- _____

Now compare what you just wrote with your positive beliefs about worry. Does worry seem worth it? If not, remind yourself of these costs when you are having a hard time detaching from your worry or feeling resistant to using your skills.

Sometimes people find themselves focusing too much on the costs of worry, leading to anxiety about the negative consequences you just identified (worry about worry). Such beliefs are called *negative metacognitions,* and understanding them is also an important part of addressing worry. We'll address those in the second section of this module.

Attention and Anxiety

One of the effects of our beliefs about worry and anxiety is that they shape how we direct our attention. To illustrate this, try this free association exercise in which you let your mind simply wander to wherever it naturally goes in response to a series of words. For each of the words in the box below, say the word out loud, close your eyes, and simply notice where your mind goes for 10 to 15 seconds, and then move on to the next word.

worry	responsibilities	health
deadline	finances	family
planning	avoidance	projects

In the space below, write down what you noticed as you did this exercise:

_____

_____

_____

_____

_____

Did you find yourself stuck in an anxious train of thought? Which words were bothersome for you? For example, the word "deadline" for Jill would likely trigger thoughts about her upcoming presentation and elicit anxiety about being able to get everything done in time. Did your mind jump to things you needed to do, or the possibility of something bad happening? If so, this is an example of the way worry directs your attention toward possible danger. These words could be associated with a lot of things, but for people who worry a lot, they're much more likely to lead to thoughts about bad things that could happen. This is because if you believe that worry can be helpful or make you feel temporarily better, your mind is going to be particularly adept at identifying possible danger.

This threat detection is necessary at some level for survival. But the words you read were just words, and don't represent any real danger. Believing that worry can be helpful, however, can make it very difficult to direct your attention away from possible threats, even if they're just words. In everyday life, you likely encounter many situations that trigger you to think about your relationships, future, health, and work. If you believe that worry is helpful for avoiding bad outcomes in any of these areas, it's also likely that you behave in a way that's vigilant to all of the possible threats, or ways in which things could turn out badly. And when you are always on the lookout for danger, you can usually find something to worry about! This hypervigilance can also drive behavior like preparing for every possible thing that could go wrong (no matter how small the chances), hyper-focusing on any negative outcomes, or constantly monitoring your thoughts and feelings, as we saw Jill doing during her dinner with friends.

Now you might have heard people say things to you like "Don't worry about it" or "Just stop worrying." You probably also know that this usually isn't helpful, and may even start to get really annoying! And you have a right to be annoyed because, paradoxically, the harder you try to suppress or block your worries, the more your worries increase and feel harder to control.

To see this for yourself, try the following exercise.

1. Close your eyes and imagine a white bear. Picture it clearly in your imagination. Imagine his fluffy white fur and large black paws. Take a few seconds to think about it and really imagine that fluffy white bear.

2. After you have a clear image of that white bear in your mind, set a timer for 1 minute. During this time, close your eyes again, and think about anything you want, *except for a white bear*. Try your best not to think about the white bear.

3. Anytime the white bear does pop in to your head, make a tally mark in the following space.

4. Ready? Set your timer for 1 minute and imagine anything except a fluffy white bear. Go!

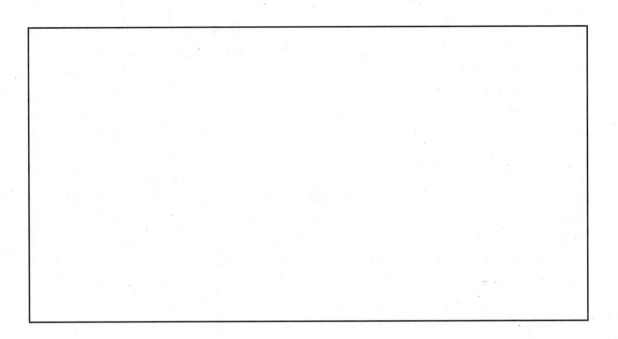

What happened? You probably thought about the white bear at least a couple times (almost everyone does). Even if you didn't think about it, you had to know you weren't thinking about it to be successful—and thus, you were thinking about it on some level of your awareness. This is an example of the paradoxical effect of thought suppression. The more you try NOT to think about something, the more you end up thinking about it!

This effect tends to be even stronger with worry thoughts. For most people, a white bear is a relatively neutral, unemotional image. But if you're trying not to think about something that makes you anxious, like something from the list of words you read earlier, it's going to be even harder to push those thoughts out of your mind. Ultimately, suppressing your thoughts just doesn't work. This is why it's not helpful when someone tells you, or you tell yourself, "Just don't worry about it!" or "Stop it!" Although this advice is well intentioned, and it may even seem reasonable to try, suppression isn't a good strategy.

Controlling Attention Through Detached Awareness

Hopefully, we've convinced you of the perils of thought suppression. You may be wondering, what is the alternative? One skill that's particularly effective is called *detached awareness*. Rather than trying to suppress or control your worries, detached awareness involves simply noticing your thoughts without responding to them. When we worry, we tend to be attached to the meaning and importance of our thoughts, and then can become consumed by them. Worry thoughts, however, are no more important than any other thoughts. They are all still just thoughts.

We'll use the detached awareness skill to apply this concept that worries are just thoughts. With detached awareness, your goal is to be a distant observer of your thoughts, simply watching them come and go. You'll try to notice your thoughts as mere thoughts, nothing more, and certainly not urgent or important messages telling you that you need to be preparing for your presentation or other things. Seeing your thoughts as simply thoughts will allow you to get some distance from them.

To help create some separation from your thoughts, it can be useful to form an image in your mind of thoughts coming and going, and below are some images that work well. The idea is to imagine placing each thought that pops into your head on some external object that passes through. For example:

1. View your thoughts and worries as trains passing through a station. Some trains are comfortable, others are noisy and dirty; some trains are really noticeable, others are easy to ignore; some trains come frequently, others less so. Thoughts can be like this, too. Rather than jumping on every train that passes through, simply watch the trains come and go, and only board the one that takes you where you want to go. Thus, instead of entertaining every single thought and worry, you only attend to the thoughts in line with what you want to focus on at that moment.

2. View your thoughts as leaves gently flowing down a stream. Picture yourself as the observer of your thoughts, sitting on the bank of the stream. Picture placing each thought on a leaf, then watch it travel downstream. Then observe the next thought come from upstream, and picture placing it on a leaf (adapted from Hayes 2005).

3. See your thoughts written on the sand, and then washed away each time the tide comes in. Observe each thought fade away as the ocean water washes over it.

To practice detached awareness, pick one of the three images, or you can create your own if you think of something that's more relatable. The more vividly you are able to imagine the thoughts coming and going, the more effective this will be. The main point is to simply create separation between you and your thoughts so that they don't control how you feel and what you do. This will be easier once you can see *worry thoughts* as just *thoughts*.

Now let's go back to the list of words you read before. Do the same exercise as earlier, reading the word out loud, then closing your eyes. However, this time, as thoughts come into your head, imagine the thoughts as trains, leaves, or writing in the sand. Observe each thought come and go, just as you would a train entering and leaving a station, leaves floating by you on a stream, or writing coming and going in the sand. You can choose to imagine a single word or a full sentence, but take your time with it. Remember, you are not trying to get rid of your thoughts or change them. Instead, you are simply observing your thoughts as mere thoughts. If the same thought comes up over and over again, that's okay. Your goal is to accept that it's there, and continue to observe it from a distance.

In the same way as before, begin by saying each word out loud while closing your eyes. Then pull up your image and notice what thoughts are produced by your mind for 10 to 15 seconds.

worry	*responsibilities*	*health*
deadline	*finances*	*family*
planning	*avoidance*	*projects*

Write what you noticed when doing this exercise, including anything that was different from the first time you read these words:

_____

_____

_____

_____

_____

Like most of the skills in this book, this exercise is difficult and takes practice, so it's okay if you didn't understand it at first. If you are like most people, you may even wonder whether you were doing it correctly. In fact, go ahead and practice observing those thoughts, too! This is a skill that takes time and only improves with practice. With practice, you'll notice an increased ability to move your attention more quickly from the anxious thoughts to other non-anxious thoughts and your ability to detach from your thoughts will improve. Ultimately, the goal is to use this technique to realize that even though you can't control which thoughts initially pop into your head, you can control and decide *how to respond* to your thoughts.

Worry Modulation Experiment

Before we finish this section of Module 4, let's return to our positive metacognitions for a moment, because beliefs that worry is helpful can also make a skill like detached awareness harder to implement in your day-to-day life. You may feel that despite the costs of worry, it still does do helpful things for you. Take a moment and think about whether you feel this might be true. To help with any doubts you might be having, we'll do an exercise called the *worry modulation experiment*. We'll compare two experiences: 1) what happens when you worry a lot, and what happens when you don't worry. By comparing the two, we can evaluate the utility of your worries. Here is how the worry modulation experiment works:

During the next week, pick one day to *maximize worry*. You are being asked to let yourself fall back into all your old habits. Don't use any of the skills that you have learned so far. Worry as much as you naturally would, and even a little more, but for only one day. The next day, do the opposite and *minimize* worry. This doesn't mean suppress anxiety and worrisome thoughts. Rather, use all the skills you've been learning to the best of your ability. This means using progressive muscle relaxation, rethinking thoughts (challenging probability overestimation and catastrophizing), and detached awareness skills as much as possible. If some worries become overwhelming, write them down and tell yourself you'll attend to them the next day. But as much as you can, use your skills, as the goal of this second day is to minimize worry by fully committing yourself to practice all of your new skills.

So what is the point of such an experiment? Well, if worry is as helpful as your positive metacognitions would lead you to believe, maximizing worry should help you be more productive, prevent bad outcomes, and lead to less anxiety. You might feel that letting go of worry, on the other hand, will cause you to neglect your responsibilities and be unproductive. The point of this exercise is to put your beliefs to the test and see whether worry is as beneficial as you once believed.

To make this clearer, let's take a look at how Jill used the worry modulation experiment. As you recall, Jill's worries increased when she remembered she had to give a presentation. Part of the reason she felt compelled to worry was because she thought that it would increase her preparedness. When Jill completed the worry modulation experiment, she was able to directly test whether worry was actually helpful.

In the first step, Jill identified what skills she'd use to minimize worry:

Worry or control behaviors to stop: *I'll let go of excessive planning and rehearsing of my presentation.*

How and when you're going to use skills: *I'll use detached awareness exercises to create more distance between myself and my worries about how the presentation will go. I'll also practice progressive muscle relaxation instead of continuing to prepare.*

Jill was concerned about what it would mean to let go of worry. She wrote down some of her feared outcomes below:

1. *I won't be prepared enough for my presentation. I'll make a lot of mistakes and my boss will be disappointed in me.*

2. *If I don't worry about the presentation, I'll probably forget to prepare for some of the follow-up questions people ask. I won't have anything to say in response, and people will think I'm incompetent.*

After specifying her fears about minimizing worry, Jill picked two days to do the experiment that were similar in terms of her other responsibilities in order to make a fair comparison of the effects of maximizing and minimizing worry. Jill also tracked her thoughts, feelings, and behaviors on each day, as well as her productivity. By comparing how these things differed across days, Jill could determine what the consequences of worry were. Let's take a look:

Increasing Worry	Minimizing Worry
Date: 4/7	Date: 4/8
Control behaviors (planned itinerary for day): Schedule time to practice and rehearse the presentation several times throughout the day.	Lack of control behaviors (make no plans): Don't rehearse or practice at all. Use my skills instead.
Thoughts: No matter how much I practice this, I feel like it isn't perfect enough.	Thoughts: When I'm not worrying about it on purpose, it doesn't seem as overwhelming to me. Detached awareness helped me get distance from my thoughts.
Feelings: Anxiety and dread, which made my heart race. When I allowed myself to focus on physical feelings, my anxiety went up more.	Feelings: Felt anxious at times about not rehearsing, but at other times I was able to enjoy the day. PMR helped me not feel as many physical symptoms like heart racing.
Productivity score for the day (Did you complete the tasks you set out to complete? Use a scale of 0–8): Productivity 4. Although I practiced the talk, I felt too overwhelmed to do any of my other chores or tasks.	Productivity score for the day (Did you complete the tasks you set out to complete? Use a scale of 0–8): Productivity 5. I didn't practice my talk, but I was able to do lots of other things like going shopping and doing my laundry.
End of day overall anxiety (0–8): 6	End of day overall anxiety (0–8): 3
Notes: Worrying makes me feel prepared, but I didn't get as much done as I would have liked.	Notes: Letting go of worry was hard, but my productivity didn't seem to suffer from minimizing worry.

Looking at Jill's experiment, we can see that worry didn't prove to be as beneficial as she thought. Even though worry made her practice more, that didn't help her feel more confident, and her anxiety ended up being more intense. Her worry-driven behaviors also took time away from getting other things done like laundry and shopping. Even though worry might have felt productive in the moment, it was overall more harmful than helpful.

Now it's your turn to test this out for yourself. Try your own worry modulation experiment by picking two days in your week that are relatively similar in terms of your responsibilities and tasks (such as two workdays). In addition, plan out what you are going to do to in order to minimize worry in the space below. There is also a worksheet at the end of the section and at http://www.newharbinger.com/44529, which you should do for home practice.

Worry or control behaviors to stop: _____

_____

_____

_____

_____

How and when you're going to use skills: _____

_____

_____

_____

_____

In addition, make some predictions about what you're afraid might happen by minimizing worry ("I won't get enough done"). We'll review these in the next section.

1. _____

_____

2. _____

_____

3. _____

_____

You should expect that minimizing worry might *feel* strange. After all, you are reversing a habit of worry that you have likely had for years. But, remember the elephants in Boston story? Remember how Fred kept banging his head against a wall because he believed that it kept the elephants out of the city? Fred never tested what would happen if he didn't keep banging his head. By conducting this experiment, you are doing what Fred never did. You are going to test out whether worry really does prevent bad things from happening or increases your productivity as much as you might think.

Section Review: Key Points

- Metacognitions are beliefs we hold about our thoughts. Worry is often caused and maintained by positive metacognitions, which are beliefs that worry is helpful in some way (for example, "Worry helps me prepare for possible bad outcomes").

- Positive metacognitions influence where you direct your attention. Specifically, believing that worry is helpful can cause you to constantly focus on things that could possibly go wrong, and have a hard time detaching from those thoughts.

- Attempting to suppress or block thoughts tends to backfire, and the suppressed thoughts arise more frequently and more strongly (remember the white bear exercise).

- Detached awareness is an effective alternative to thought suppression. Rather than trying to push away a thought or change it, detached awareness involves simply noticing the thought from a distance and letting it pass. This reduces the control the thought holds on your attention, and can help you decide how to respond to your thoughts.

Home Practice

- **Detached Awareness:** Practice detached awareness each day, logging how it went in the form on the next page and at http://www.newharbinger.com/44529. You can keep practicing with the list of words used before, but eventually move to using it in day-to-day situations that trigger anxiety.

- **Worry Modulation Experiment:** Pick one day to maximize worry, and one day to minimize worry. Plan out how you're going to minimize worry and identify your predictions about the outcome of the two days in the space provided earlier in the section. Review how each day went in the form on the next page and at http://www.newharbinger.com/44529.

- **Keep Using Your Skills:** The more you practice cognitive restructuring and progressive muscle relaxation, the more automatic these skills will become, and the closer you'll get to overcoming your anxiety.

Detached Awareness Log

Remember, detached awareness isn't about avoiding thoughts. Instead, we're trying to notice the thought, avoid escalating the reaction to it, and view the event as an observer, instead of as the person experiencing it. Below, log your practice of detached awareness and how successfully you were able to objectively notice and observe your thoughts.

Date	Describe the situation in which you practiced detached awareness.	How successful were you at objectively observing your thoughts?	Comments

Worry Modulation Experiment

Use the form below to guide you in evaluating how each day of your worry modulation experiment goes.

Increasing Worry	Minimizing Worry
Date:	Date:
Control behaviors (planned itinerary for day):	Lack of control behaviors (make no plans):
Thoughts:	Thoughts:
Feelings:	Feelings:
Productivity score for the day (Did you complete the tasks you set out to complete? Use a scale of 0–8):	Productivity score for the day (Did you complete the tasks you set out to complete? Use a scale of 0–8):
End of day overall anxiety (0–8):	End of day overall anxiety (0–8):
Notes:	Notes:

SECTION II

Worry Postponement

In this next section, we'll go over negative metacognitions in more depth, as well introduce another skill that can help you get out of the cycle of anxiety, which we call worry time. But first, we're going to use the results of your worry modulation experiment to highlight another important point about worry.

Reviewing Your Experiment

In the "Detached Awareness Module," you made some predictions about what would happen if you minimized worry. Let's take a look at those briefly. In the example provided, Jill thought that if she didn't let herself worry on the day leading up to her presentation, she'd make a lot of mistakes and be unprepared for follow-up questions. See how she evaluated those predictions afterward.

Situation: *Using skills to minimize worry leading up to a work presentation*	
Prediction	**Actual Outcome**
1. I won't be prepared enough for my presentation. I'll make a lot of mistakes and my boss will be disappointed in me.	1. I made one mistake, but no one said anything about it. My boss said I did a good job.
2. If I don't worry about the presentation, I'll probably forget to prepare for some of the follow-up questions people ask. I won't have anything to say in response, and people will think I'm incompetent.	2. There was one follow-up question I wasn't prepared for, but I was able to think on my feet and give a decent answer. It's unlikely that preparing more would have helped me come up with a better answer anyway.

Even though it was a bit nerve-wracking for Jill to minimize her worry on the day leading up to the presentation, it turned out that her predictions about things going poorly as a result didn't come true. Her boss said she did a good job, and she was able to answer follow-up questions after the presentation despite not preparing as much as she usually does. Letting go of worry didn't have the negative consequences that she feared.

Although her concerns didn't fully come true, you may have noticed that things didn't go perfectly for Jill on her presentation. For this reason, it's important to *evaluate outcomes as objectively as possible.* Jill did make a mistake on her presentation, and her instinct was to focus on that as a sign that she should have prepared more. Her prediction, however, was that she'd "make a lot of mistakes and her boss would be disappointed in her," which clearly was not what happened. To help stay objective and keep the big picture in mind, it can be useful to use the skills you learned in Module 3 for challenging your thoughts. For instance, Jill could evaluate the evidence for and against the idea that her boss would be disappointed in her (see Step 2 of "Challenging Probability Overestimation"). The evidence for this idea includes the fact that she made one mistake, whereas the evidence against it was that no one seemed to notice the mistake, and her boss said she did a good job. She could also use her challenging catastrophic thinking skills to evaluate the actual severity of any negative outcomes (*so what* that she wasn't prepared for one follow-up question?) and how she coped with such outcomes (she thought of a decent answer on the spot) (see Steps 2 and 3 of "Challenging Catastrophic Thinking").

With this example in mind, in the table below, review your own predictions about what would happen if you minimized your worry. When evaluating the actual outcome, check whether you are being objective about the outcome and keeping the big picture in mind. Use your skills for challenging thoughts as necessary.

Situation: *Using skills to minimize worry*	
Prediction	**Actual Outcome**
1.	1.
2.	2.

How Accurate Is Your Worry?

The previous exercise is an illustration of the idea that although it often *feels* important to listen to our worries, they're not always accurate. We discussed this in terms of your beliefs about worry specifically, but it's an important idea to consider for any worry that might come up for you. Worry sends the strong message that something bad *could* happen, but how often does that bad outcome *actually* happen?

When considering that question, many people with anxiety will immediately think of a time in their past when something bad did occur (a poor presentation, someone got sick). These negative events tend to stand out in our memories, which makes some sense because that helps us learn from them. What doesn't usually stick out in our memories, however, is all the times when we were worried about something that did *not* happen. Again, this makes sense, as there isn't much reason to remember the absence of a negative outcome. But it can cause our minds to be biased toward thinking that bad outcomes happen all the time, because those are things we focus our attention on.

To counter this, you'll be doing what we call a worry contrast exercise, where you contrast what your worry predicts is going to happen in a given situation with the actual outcome, just like you did earlier with your beliefs about worry. Then you'll answer whether your worry prediction was in fact accurate, using your challenging questions skills to answer as objectively as possible. It can be helpful to do this a number of times to gather more data about the accuracy of your worry, so you'll also do this for home practice using the worksheet at the end of this module. For now, start by looking at the examples below from your workbook companions, and then try to think of a past worry where you can evaluate whether your feared outcome occurred. It may be helpful to look at past home practice worksheets to identify a testable worry prediction.

Worry Prediction	Actual Outcome	Was Your Worry Accurate? *Evaluate evidence for and against and de-catastrophize to answer*
(Elijah) This paper is terrible, I'm going to get a poor grade and have to retake the class.	Got a B-	Not really. It was not a great grade, but it wasn't terrible, and it doesn't actually put me at risk of failing the class.
(Sofia) My son said he was going to be home an hour ago; he must have gotten in an accident.	His basketball practice went late, and then he had to drop off a friend. Everything was fine.	Not at all.
(Jill) Our client is upset with me because I was slow to respond to her emails last week. We might lose her business and I'll be responsible.	She seemed rather curt in subsequent emails, but then she brought up another project she wanted to hire us for.	No. She may have been annoyed, I can't say for sure, but it clearly was not a big deal because she wants to keep working with us.

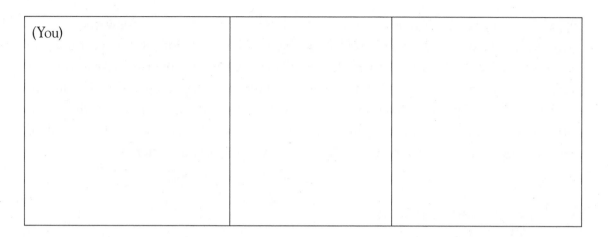

(You)		

In the examples provided, notice how even though the actual outcome was not always totally positive, the prediction was always exaggerated. Elijah was not thrilled about his grade, but it was not the catastrophe his worry predicted. Jill didn't have clear evidence about whether the client was upset or not ("seeming curt" isn't particularly objective evidence), but she did know definitively that they weren't losing the client. Rather, her office was going to be hired for another job. So when evaluating the outcomes related to your own worry predictions, be sure to pay attention to the actual predictions made and whether you are considering all the evidence in an objective manner.

Hopefully at this point you are starting to realize that *worry isn't a reliable predictor of the future.* This can be a helpful thing to remind yourself of when you're having a hard time letting go of a worry thought, and as you do more worry contrast exercises this will become more evident.

Before we move on though, we should address two final points. First, you may notice yourself thinking something like, "Sure, the bad outcome didn't happen, but that's because I did something to prevent it. My worry helped me take action!" If that's the case for you, it's important to remember our distinction between worry and problem solving (discussed in Module 1, Section II). Worry is an unhelpful *thinking* response to a potential problem. It involves taking something we're anxious about and spinning it around in our head rather than taking action. If you took active steps to prevent a bad outcome, then good work—you may have been problem solving! But that doesn't necessarily mean worry was responsible for preventing a bad outcome. It's also important to ask yourself whether you *know* that the bad outcome would have occurred if you hadn't done something to prevent it (remember the elephants in Boston story). This idea will be discussed further in Module 6.

A final note is that sometimes worry can cause what is called a *self-fulfilling prophecy.* This means that the negative impacts of worry can lead the worry prediction to become true. This happens a lot for Elijah when doing work for his classes. He worries about doing poorly on an assignment, this worry leads him to avoid doing the work and have difficulty concentrating on it, and as a result he ends up getting a poor grade. These types of situations can make it seem like worry is an accurate predictor of the future, but it's important to keep in mind that self-fulfilling prophecies tend to happen when we don't have the skills to cope with our worry. Now that you've learned some tools to manage anxiety, you can use them to prevent the worry cycle from taking over, and prove to yourself that your worry thoughts are not so accurate after all.

Negative Metacognitions

We've spent a good portion of the last section and a half challenging the idea that worry is helpful or accurate. On the flip side of this, however, are *negative metacognitions*, which refer to beliefs about worry being uncontrollable and leading to disastrous consequences. These beliefs cause problems because they often lead us to start worrying *about* worry, which amplifies anxiety and often leads to ineffective behavior, such as avoidance.

For example, when Sofia thinks about returning to work after being a stay-at-home mom for many years, she gets anxious about how much worry would interfere with her ability to do the job well. She thinks: "I won't be able to control my worry when I have all the responsibilities and pressure of a real job. My worry will spiral out of control and I'll panic!" As a result, she avoids returning to work, even though she'd really like to do so. She also misses out on the chance to see whether her beliefs about the uncontrollability and disastrous consequences of worry are actually true. Her negative metacognitions, therefore, keep her stuck in a cycle of worry and avoidance.

Negative metacognitions can also intensify anxiety when we start to worry. Elijah, for example, often experiences anxiety when taking tests. Although this is a normal reaction, it becomes more of a problem when he becomes convinced that his anxiety is going to significantly affect his exam performance, especially his ability to concentrate and remember important information. As a result, when he takes a test and starts to notice himself worrying, he begins catastrophizing about his worry, thinking, "I'm so anxious for this test; this is really going to screw me over. There is no way I'm going to be able to control my worry, and I'm not going to be able to focus or remember what I need to. I'm done for!"

You can probably imagine the effect that this sort of thinking has: Elijah's anxiety continues to increase as he keeps telling himself he's not going to be able to do well on the test if he's anxious, and he spends just as much time thinking about his anxiety as he does on the test questions. Ultimately, Elijah's negative beliefs about the disastrous consequences of worry cause relatively normal levels of anxiety on a test to turn into a spiral of worry and a poor performance on the exam.

Before we start talking about how to combat such negative metacognitions about worry, do a brief self-assessment on some of the beliefs you might hold related to the negative consequences of worry. Check off any of the beliefs from the list below (adapted from Wells and Cartwright-Hatton 2004) that apply to you, and write any additional negative beliefs you have about the negative consequences of worry or your ability to control it.

Common Negative Metacognitions

☐ My worrying thoughts persist, no matter how I try to stop them.

☐ When I start worrying, I can't stop.

☐ I could make myself sick with worrying.

☐ I can't ignore my worrying thoughts.

☐ My worrying could make me go mad.

☐ My worrying is dangerous for me.

☐ Other: _____

☐ Other: _____

☐ Other: _____

Now think to yourself about how these beliefs impact your worry. Do they increase your anxiety when you're feeling anxious? Do they cause you to avoid things you'd otherwise like to do because you feel like you won't be able to control your worry? Even if you don't immediately realize it, the answer to these questions is often yes for individuals with high levels of anxiety, so read on about how to combat such beliefs.

Interrupting Worry

In order to better understand whether worry is truly uncontrollable, imagine the following scenario:

You are home by yourself and you are worrying. Your mind is totally occupied by your anxious thoughts, your body is tense, your breathing is shallow, and you can feel your heart beating as you pace around your house thinking about everything you have to do. Then all of a sudden, the doorbell rings. You go to answer it and it's a close friend of yours that you haven't seen in a year.

What happens to your worry in this scenario? It goes down, right? In fact, it probably completely goes away, at least momentarily. No longer are you intently focused on your worries; instead, you've shifted your attention to the friend at the door.

Now what if instead of your friend at the door, you received a phone call saying a family member is in the hospital and that you should come immediately. What happens to your attention then? Are you still worried about how much you have to do, or are you focused on getting to the hospital so you can be there for your family member?

In both of these scenarios, you are likely to shift your attention to what is going on around you, and in doing so you are exerting control over your worry. Such situations illustrate that you actually do have enough control over your worry to stop your anxious thoughts and engage with the situation around you. This is easier to do when something really important comes up, but the same principle applies for any time we're worrying: *our worry is influenced by where we choose to direct our attention.* For example, think back to your detached awareness skill, where you learned to observe your thoughts, including worry thoughts, from a distance. This was another example of your ability to control worry by deciding whether and how to shift your attention. Worry may *feel* uncontrollable, but it can always be interrupted by refocusing your attention.

Choosing to Worry

Let's do another activity to illustrate the impact that attention has on our worrying. For this exercise, prepare an alarm to go off in one minute. During this minute, you are going to worry as much as you can. Take all the things you are stressed and worried about and run them around and around in your head. Ready? Set your alarm, and go worry!

[Let one minute pass.]

Okay, worry time is over. What happened? Were you able to make yourself worry? For most people, especially those who often are anxious, the answer is a resounding yes! This exercise, while not particularly fun, illustrates how worry can be controlled. You made a choice to worry. By focusing your attention on all the things that might go wrong in your life, you were able to increase your worry. This actually mirrors what we often do in our lives when worry takes over. It may not always feel like it, but we *choose* to worry. In response to an anxious thought, we decide to let our attention slip toward worry and away from other ways of responding to that thought or the situation around us.

This idea isn't meant to place blame on ourselves for worrying. Controlling worry is hard, especially when it's a pattern of thinking that's well practiced. Rather, the idea that we choose to worry can also be empowering. If we choose to worry, we can also choose *not* to worry. We can choose to direct our attention elsewhere, and break the worry cycle. In fact, if you are reading these words, you just did that! A minute ago you were worrying, and then when your alarm went off, you chose to refocus your attention on this page and continued reading. Yes, the alarm helped, but you also could have kept worrying, and instead decided to come back to your workbook. The main message here is that, although we can't control whether an anxious thought comes up, *we do have control over how we respond to our thoughts.* Reminding ourselves of this can help us challenge our negative beliefs about worry being something out of our control that has disastrous consequences.

Worry Postponement

So how can we capitalize on this insight that we have control over our response to anxious thoughts? One skill that can be quite helpful is called *worry postponement*. This involves picking a specific 30-minute period during the day when you are *allowed* to worry. The catch is that all other worries that come up during your day need to be postponed to that designated "worry time."

Why is this helpful? First, consolidating your worry into a specific part of the day gives you the freedom to focus on more important things throughout the rest of your day. In addition, it can be a helpful way to prove to yourself that you *can* actually control your worries enough to postpone them to a later time. If a worry feels really important and is hard to shake, it can be a little bit easier to redirect your attention if you've told yourself you can worry about it later. Over time, postponing your worry will increase your confidence in your ability to control your worry and give you more practice in shifting attention away from your anxious thoughts.

Another reason why worry postponement works is that oftentimes when people get to their designated "worry time," they either forgot what they were planning to worry about or it no longer seems so important. Worry thoughts can often seem extremely urgent and important in the moment, but with some time and distance from them, their significance decreases. So when you get to your worry time, you don't *need* to worry if you no longer feel compelled to. You simply *allow* yourself to worry if it still feels relevant.

If you catch yourself worrying outside of the worry time, or are unsure of whether you are just worrying or responding to a real problem, the first question to ask yourself is: "Do I need to solve this problem right now?" Usually the answer is no. But if it's an urgent issue, then go ahead and problem solve (take active steps toward a solution), rather than worrying about it. If it can wait, however, then postpone your concern to worry time, and instead refocus your attention on whatever is most important in that moment. Or if you are worrying about something that you need to take care of in the near future, make a plan for when you'll problem solve, and then redirect your focus on the present. This process is illustrated in the figure below to help you decide what to do.

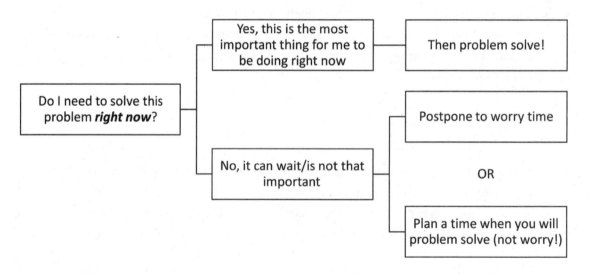

Figure 4.1. *Worry Postponement Decision Tree*

To see what this process looks like in more depth, look at the Worry Postponement Log from Elijah (you'll do this for home practice using the worksheet at the end of this module).

Worry Postponement Log

Planned Worry Time: 7:00 to 7:30 p.m.

Day & Time	Worry Thought	Intensity (0–10) in the moment	Do I need to solve this now? If yes, then do it. If no, then postpone or plan.	Intensity (0–10) during worry time
Tuesday, 1 a.m.	Rent is due next week, my credit card balance keeps growing, and I don't even know how much money I have in my bank account.	7	No, sleep is more important. I'll take a look at my finances tomorrow evening and make a plan.	4. I'm still anxious about finances, but not as much as last night and it helps to have a plan.
Wednesday, 10 a.m.	The paper I turned in last week was terrible and I'm going to get a bad grade for the class.	6	No, I should focus on this class that I'm in.	5. I'm still kind of anxious about my grade, but at least I didn't spend the whole time in class worrying about it.
Wednesday, 4 p.m.	My professor hasn't responded to my email; he probably thinks I don't deserve to be in this class.	6	No, I should focus my energy on my workout right now.	1. Seems like a pretty silly concern now.

As you can see, Elijah's worries about finances reflect a real problem that needs addressing, but not in the middle of the night. So he made a plan for when he'd take care of the issue, which helped him control his worry. When worry time came around, he was still a bit anxious about it, but not nearly as much as the night before. Another one of his worries, which was about the paper he'd turned in, was still a concern at worry time. However, by postponing his thinking about it, he was able to focus better in class earlier in the day. Finally, the worry about his professor's lack of email response ended up seeming totally irrational to him later that day, so delaying that worry was especially helpful.

Section Review: Key Points

- Worry isn't an accurate predictor of future outcomes. One helpful way to demonstrate this to yourself is to track the predictions your worry makes about the future and compare them with actual outcomes.

- Negative metacognitions are beliefs that worry is uncontrollable or leads to disastrous consequences. Such beliefs can lead to unhelpful avoidance of potentially stressful situations, or amplify worry when you do feel anxious.

- Although worry sometimes feels uncontrollable, it can be interrupted by redirecting your attention to what is going on in the present moment. Because you can choose where to focus your attention, you can exert control over worry.

- Postponing your worry to a specific period of time in the day ("worry time") can help free space throughout your day to focus on the things you most care about. Often, when "worry time" comes around, earlier worries no longer seem so important.

Home Practice

- **Worry Contrast Exercise:** When you notice you are worrying about something, write down what your worry is predicting will happen in the Worry Contrast Worksheet (also available at http://www.newharbinger.com/44529). Later, evaluate how the actual outcome compared to your prediction. You can also do this retrospectively.

- **Worry Postponement:** Choose a 20- to 30-minute period of each day (not immediately before bedtime) when you'll allow yourself to worry. All other worries during the day should be postponed to that time. Use the Worry Postponement Log (also available at http://www.newharbinger.com/44529) to track how the intensity of your worry changes after you delay it to worry time, and to sort through whether worries represent pressing issues that need to be problem solved immediately or can wait for another time.

- **Keep Using Your Skills:** Continue using PMR, challenging beliefs, and detached awareness skills as needed to respond effectively to your anxiety.

Worry Contrast Worksheet

Worry Prediction	Actual Outcome	Was Your Worry Accurate? *Evaluate evidence for and against and de-catastrophize to answer*

Worry Postponement Log

Scheduled Worry Time: _____

Day & Time	Worry Thought	Intensity (0–10) in the moment	Do I need to solve this now? If yes, then do it. If no, then postpone or plan.	Intensity (0–10) during worry time

MODULE 5

Facing Feared Scenarios and Images

The last two modules focused on tools that help you challenge and gain distance from worry thoughts. In the next two modules, you'll learn about the benefits of confronting your fears head-on, and how to do so effectively. But first, let's talk a bit more about worry. As discussed earlier, worry is an unhelpful *thinking* response to a potential problem that emphasizes negative interpretations of a scenario. Worry tends to be *verbal* in nature. That is, most of your worries come to you in the form of words and sentences used to process an event that could have a negative outcome. Although language can be your friend, it can also be used as a weapon against you when it comes to anxiety. This is because processing scary situations in an overly verbal way can function as a form of avoidance.

Think about it this way. What sounds more difficult: using language to think about your worst-case scenario or watching a movie of it happening in vivid detail? Most people would say the movie is much more difficult, as the vivid visuals and sound effects bring up much stronger emotions. So, when the thought of a negative scenario comes up for us, using language to worry is a natural response to protect ourselves from facing the full image of a feared outcome. It helps you avoid experiencing the full intensity of your feared scenario. Now it becomes easy to see that *worry is avoidance!* Let's consider Sofia:

Sofia recently learned that her older son will be taking a trip during his college spring break to New Orleans. Although happy for her son, she asked him to call her every day during his trip for reassurance that he was okay. However, the day her son flew to New Orleans, she didn't hear from him. Sofia tried to challenge her catastrophic thinking using detached awareness, but when she still hadn't heard from him the day after the flight, she gave in to her urge to search anxiously for any sign that he made it there safely. She desperately searched online to make sure there were no reports of an airplane accident. Automatic thoughts popped into her mind, such as "What if the plane crashed and the authorities don't even know yet? Maybe he ended up in the hospital after drinking too much!" With uncertainty lingering in her mind, it was relatively easy for Sofia to imagine the worst-case scenarios and potential catastrophes. Sofia felt like she couldn't tolerate these scary images, and told herself that she must have reassurance that he was okay to avoid these catastrophic images taking over her thinking. As soon as afternoon arrived with still no word from her son, Sofia sent him a long string of text messages and called him repeatedly until he finally picked up. She was relieved of course to hear that her son was okay and just forgot to call her, but she was upset with herself that she'd wasted so much time being on edge.

Sofia was worried. I'm sure you can relate to her. Worry can feel productive in the short term, yet it never seems to address our underlying fears and anxiety in a meaningful way. What can we do about this? Well, we can use principles from *exposure therapy* to target worry thoughts. Traditionally, therapists use exposure therapy to help people overcome phobias by making them encounter their fears in person. People with a spider phobia might be required to first look at pictures of spiders, then look at a spider in a glass jar, and finally hold a live spider in their hand. Teaching people to approach their fears instead of avoiding them allows them to learn that the feared situations are actually safe. This is an extremely important idea, but a hard one for people to fully buy in to sometimes, so let's dive in a little more.

Why Face Your Fears?

When we encounter a feared situation, or sometimes even think about one, we're faced with two basic possibilities: face the fear or avoid it. As discussed previously, avoidance doesn't just mean avoiding the situation; it can also involve things like seeking reassurance, over-preparing, or undertaking other tasks with the purpose of avoiding anxiety. Avoidance often feels better in the short term, but it has significant costs. Let's track the consequences of avoidance below.

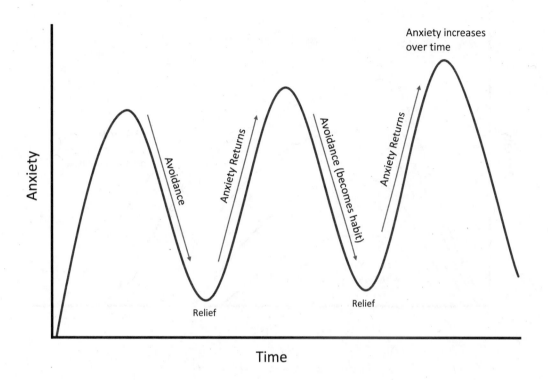

Figure 5.1. *Avoidance Model of Anxiety*

As you can see, avoidance reduces our anxiety temporarily. But what happens the next time you encounter that situation or thought? The fear spikes right back up again. You can continue to avoid each time, but the fear will come back every time you encounter the situation. In fact, avoiding tends to make the fear get even worse. This is because by avoiding, you are basically telling your brain that the situation is, in fact, dangerous. For example, when Sofia constantly texts her son for reassurance of his safety, it makes her feel like he's not safe unless he's responded saying he's okay. Furthermore, the relief provided by avoidance also feels good (at least relative to not avoiding), and therefore becomes a habit.

Now let's look at what happens when you face your fears on the next graph.

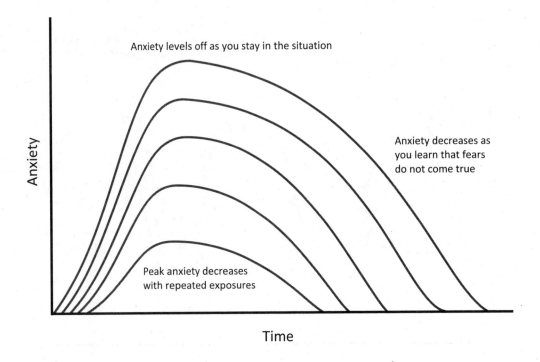

Figure 5.2. *Exposure Model of Anxiety*

In this case, you encounter a feared scenario, your anxiety goes up, but you don't avoid it. What do you think will happen? Well, the anxiety will continue to go up, but it doesn't go up indefinitely. Eventually it will level off, and then even begin to go down. By itself, this might not look that much better than avoiding. However, if you approach that feared situation a second time, things get better. Specifically, the peak of the fear is lower, and the anxiety reduces more over the course of the exposure. Do it repeatedly, and eventually the fear response becomes minimal and you'll no longer feel the urge to avoid.

Why does this happen? Well, when you repeatedly face a feared situation rather than avoid it, you get the opportunity to see that the things you're afraid of don't actually happen, or are not as bad as you feared. Essentially, your brain realizes that the alarm system going off is a false alarm, and that you're not actually in danger. In addition, you get a chance to see that the anxiety you're experiencing is tolerable and harmless, rather than something to avoid at all costs. By experiencing these things, your automatic fear response gradually subsides.

Facing Worst-Case Scenarios

There are two ways that exposure techniques can be applied to you. One is to face real-life situations or things that you fear. This is called *behavioral exposure,* and we'll go over it in Module 6. A second way to use exposure is to confront worst-case scenarios in your mind using imagery (imagery exposure).

Imagining your worst-case scenario likely sounds quite difficult, but we promise that it can have some very powerful effects. Leaning in to your worst fears by vividly imagining them gives you the opportunity to learn that the associated distress isn't as unmanageable as your anxiety makes it out to be. You learn that the image of a feared scenario is just that—an image. Because these thoughts are not real situations, your mind will get used to them and the distress will decrease, just like in the graph above. Over time, the worries and worry-driven behaviors that stem from these worst-case scenarios decrease in intensity as well.

This skill is quite different than all the others we've practiced up to this point. The skills you've used so far—learning to relax physically, rethinking your thoughts—have all been targeted at reducing your anxiety much like taking medication if you have the flu. Imagery exposure, however, is like getting a flu vaccine rather than taking the medicine when you're already sick. Getting a vaccine doesn't treat the symptoms you are having in the moment but rather boosts your immunity to the flu (or these worries and anxiety, in our case) for the long term. This is initially very challenging but with practice you'll see a significant reduction in your anxiety in the long term.

Why Do Images Help?

This is a fair question to ask! It can be hard to believe that worries will just go away by using your imagination to visualize the scariest things possible. A lot of people even expect that it will make their worries increase. Although this concern is certainly understandable, there are specific reasons why imagery is helpful and brings us closer to letting go of avoidance.

Remember, worry is a language-based process. It relies on words and sentences to represent your fear so you don't have to encounter it in full color. Instead of avoiding those images with our language-based worries (or other forms of avoidance), imagery exposure will help you approach these images and conquer your fears. Because images prevent you from using language as an avoidance technique, you'll have a better chance to learn whether your biggest fear is really so intolerable.

Practicing Visualization

Before jumping into imagery exposures, it's important to practice visualization so you can better immerse yourself in the exercises you'll be doing later. Successful visualization requires both high levels of vividness and sustained attention, and you might realize you respond to certain elements of visualization more easily than others. We'll start with imagining neutral scenes so you can get the hang of it before imagining more unpleasant scenarios.

Read the script below and visualize the scene in as much detail as possible. Once you read it, close your eyes and use your imagination to immerse yourself in this world as best as you can. Really try to feel like you are there:

> *You are sitting on the bank of a bubbling river. Right near the river is a cliff from which a waterfall pours over the rocky ledge into the pool of water below. The sound of the water bouncing on the rocks makes a gurgling noise, and mist from the waterfall lands on your face. You can feel the cool dampness on your skin and smell the salt in the air. The sunshine illuminates the clouds of mist, and you can see the water shimmer like specks of gold.*

1. Rate how *vivid* the scene was on a scale of 0 (no image) to 100 (feels like you were there).

   _____

2. How many times did your attention wander away from the scene?

   _____

3. Which part of the scene was easiest to imagine?

   _____

   _____

4. Which part of the scene was difficult to imagine?

   _____

   _____

If you had any difficulty visualizing this scene, remember that visualization is a skill that takes practice. Also, if some elements of the scene (sight, sound, touch) stood out to you, you can focus more on those to make the scene more vivid. These will also be important for when you create your own scene. If this was difficult, practice a few more times to try and increase your ability to visualize. You can also find an additional visualization exercise at http://www.newhar binger.com/44529.

Imagery Exposure

Now that you've had some practice with visualization exercises, it's time to figure out what you'll be imagining. The first step is to identify the worst-case feared scenario that underlies your most frequent and bothersome worries. Often our day-to-day worries bother us much because if they came true, it feels like it would mean something much more significant and catastrophic. We can think of these underlying concerns as *core fears*. For example, people who worry a lot about every single purchase they make might have an underlying fear that they will bring their family to financial ruin by overspending, and as a result the family will become homeless. Other underlying fears might be things like contracting a serious illness and missing out on a chance to live a fulfilling life, or doing so poorly in school that you are expelled from college and your career prospects are completely ruined.

Once we have a sense of the core fear underlying a worry domain, we can then make the fears more concrete by asking, "What would it look like if this were to come true?"

Let's look at some additional examples from your workbook companions.

Sofia

Worry Theme: *My son's safety*

Underlying Fear: *Something devastating will happen to my older son and it will be my fault because I didn't look out for his safety enough.*

Worst-Case Scenario: *My son doesn't call me during his vacation because he drank too much and ended up in the hospital. People blame me for letting him go on vacation in a new city unsupervised.*

Elijah

Worry Theme: *School performance*

Underlying Fear: *I'll never be able to finish school or accomplish anything meaningful because of my anxiety and procrastination. I'll be seen as a failure and no one will want to be in a relationship with me.*

Worst-Case Scenario: *I fail the assignment I've procrastinated on, and my graduate advisor informs me that I'll be forced to leave school. Because I don't have a degree, I can't pay off all my debt and my girlfriend leaves.*

For each of the examples above, you can see how a daily worry theme isn't just about the core worry, but connects to a much bigger concern. For Sofia, her concern about her son is driven by the fear that she will be responsible for anything that happens to him. For Elijah, his worry about school connects to a fear that failure means he will lose his relationship. Imagining these worst-case scenarios may seem a bit cruel, but using imagery exposure to make the underlying concern less terrifying can help take a lot of the power away from the daily worries. Imagery exposure gets at the source of the fear, rather than the surface of it, which is why it's one of the most powerful tools you can use.

Your Worst-Case Scenarios

Now let's turn to your worst-case scenarios. Start by choosing a common worry theme, and then identify the underlying fear by going to the end of your chain of worries and asking yourself, "What is the worst thing that could happen?" or "What would be so bad about this?" You might have to ask yourself this several times to get to the heart of it. This is similar to the questions you asked yourself when identifying catastrophic thinking, but this time you're not trying to challenge these thoughts. Rather, try to think about what it would mean to you if this worst-case scenario came true, as this will help get at the underlying fear. Often the meaning will be about things like being a failure, living an unfulfilling life, missing out on important things, or being responsible for others' pain. We recognize these are tough things to think about, but we promise it's a powerful tool, so stay with it!

Once you have a sense of the underlying fear, make it more specific by thinking about a concrete image or scene that captures this worst-case scenario coming true, in the same way that your workbook companions did above. These may even be frightening images that have popped into your mind in the past, but that you've tried to push out because they were too scary. You don't have to elaborate too much on the scenario at this point, as you'll fill in the details later. Try to come up with three different scenarios below, though you may realize that some of your worries have the same underlying fear.

Worry Theme	Underlying Fear	Worst-Case Scenario

Creating an Imagery Exposure Script

Once you have your worst-case scenarios, it's time to make a script to help you vividly imagine the scene. This is like writing a scene in a movie that describes a couple minutes of action. Here are some guidelines for making the script most effective:

1. Write in the first-person, using "I."

2. Write in the present tense (for example, "I'm coming home from work…").

3. Use sensory details to help fill out the scene:

    a.   Physical feelings of anxiety or other emotions (for example, heart racing)

    b.   Detailed images of surroundings

    c.   Other senses (sounds, smells, touch)

4. *Do not* simply list worried thoughts that you'd have in the scene (such as "I worry about what I will do for money?"). Remember, we're trying to go beyond a verbal way of describing anxiety in order to create an image.

5. Try to get at the *meaning* of the event (for example, "This means I have failed").

Let's look at a sample script for Sofia to give you a better sense of how this works:

I'm sitting at home paying some bills in my living room when I get a phone call from a number in New Orleans. My heart instantly starts racing and I stand up in anticipation of news about my older son. I pick up and it's a nurse who tells me he's been admitted to the hospital for alcohol poisoning. She tells me his stomach is being pumped and he's not in great shape. My stomach drops and I sink into the couch in my living room. I can hardly speak I'm so upset. After providing the details of his condition, the nurse says in a stern voice, "I know that I wouldn't let my college-age son go to New Orleans alone; you should really keep a closer eye on him." My body surges with anxiety when she says that. This is all my fault. I should never have let him go. I'm such an irresponsible mother. I feel weak, fragile, and disoriented, and I drop the phone that's in my hand. I look at a picture of my older son on the table next to me, seeing his smiling face, and feel overwhelmed with regret and shame.

This is a tough scene to imagine, but there are some details that make it really effective. For one, it creates a scene Sofia can really imagine by describing details of her environment (the living room, the picture of her son). It also describes her bodily sensations (heart racing, stomach dropping) and behaviors (sinking into the couch, dropping the phone). Finally, the scene makes the meaning of the worst-case scenario very salient. Rather than just a tragic event happening to her son, the nurse suggests that Sofia has been irresponsible, which triggers her underlying fear that she's responsible for any harm.

Your Script

For your first script, look back at your worst-case scenarios and pick the one that you expect to be the least distressing. It's best to start with a slightly easier one because it allows you to gain mastery in learning the procedures and details of imagery exposure at lower levels of distress, which makes it more likely that you'll be successful in effectively using imagery exposure for your biggest fear.

In the space below, write a scene capturing your worst-case scenario (don't start visualizing yet). Follow the guidelines outlined above, and use Sofia's scene as an example. Make sure your worst-case scenario is something you can realistically imagine happening, or it won't be effective. We realize that even writing this out can be upsetting, but this is the first step toward overcoming your fears through exposure.

Scene 1: _____

_____

_____

_____

_____

_____

_____

_____

_____

_____

_____

_____

_____

Steps for Imagery Exposure

Good work writing your first imagery exposure script! If you are feeling apprehensive about going forward with this, remember that by doing these exposure exercises and facing your fears repeatedly, the emotional distress will decrease over time and the image will be just an image. By facing these feared images, you'll be able to change the meaning that image has, which will take away the power that these fears have over you.

Please use the steps below to guide you through the imagery exposure. This procedure for imagery exposure is derived from evidence-based treatment guidelines (Craske and Barlow 2006). It's best to try this out in a comfortable environment where there will be no distractions. Please get a timer or watch beforehand so you can set a five-minute alarm for Step 4.

1. Read the description of the image, then close your eyes and imagine the scene as if it were happening now. Focus on the details of the scene that make it most vivid to you (your physical feelings, what you see, what you hear, its personal meaning to you).

2. After about 30 seconds, rate the vividness of the image and your distress level using the subjective units of distress scale (SUDS) below.

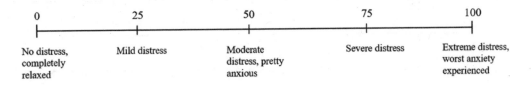

Figure 5.3. *Subjective Units of Distress Scale (SUDS)*

Subjective units of distress scale (SUDS): _____

Vividness from 0 (no image) to 100 (feels like you are there): _____

3. If the image is unclear or you rate it at less than 50 on the vividness scale, spend another minute or two imagining the event in the present tense as a participant rather than as an observer. You may also want to add more sensory details to the script to make it more vivid (what you see, hear, and feel).

4. Once you have a vivid image that's emotionally evocative (produces anxiety greater than 50 on the SUDS), observe the image for five minutes. Set a timer to let you know

when the five-minute period is up so you are not watching the clock as you do the exposure. As you imagine the event, let yourself experience any emotions produced by the image. Don't try to change either the image you see or what you are experiencing emotionally or physically. The most important thing is to let yourself fully face the image and the anxiety. Rate your SUDS level again.

Post-imagery SUDS: _____

5. After completing five minutes of imagery exposure, ask yourself the following questions:

- Because I imagined this event, will it actually happen?

- What are the actual odds that this will occur?

- If this event were to happen, what resources would I have to cope with the outcome?

- How would I cope a month later, several months, a year, and even ten years later?

- Am I over-magnifying the meaning of this imagined situation?

The goal of asking these questions is to foster your more realistic thinking strategies learned previously in this book and to recognize that it's just an image rather than fact. Not all of these will necessarily be helpful, so just focus on the ones that are.

Reviewing Your Exposure and Next Steps

First of all, congratulate yourself on doing one of the scariest things you could be asked to do! Hopefully, you got used to the image at least a little bit over the course of the exposure and saw your SUDS rating decrease. If not, don't be discouraged. As with everything you've learned so far, imagery exposure requires repetition, and it can take a few repetitions for anxiety to go significantly down.

Second, it's important to make sure you are doing the exposures correctly. Ask yourself whether are you using any avoidance behaviors during the imagery exposure, such as distracting yourself, not imagining the hardest parts of the image, or changing the scene so there is a more favorable outcome. Thinking about the questions in Step 5 ("What are the odds?") during imagery exposure can even be avoidance, so don't go to that step early. If you notice any avoidance, remind yourself to stick with the feared image, including the hardest parts, for the duration of the exercise. Remember your vividness should be at least 50 out of 100.

This next week you should keep doing exposures to the worst-case scenario you just imagined until it no longer produces much distress. The goal is to get bored with the image. You can keep track of your progress on the Imagery Exposure Recording Form at the end of the module and at http://www.newharbinger.com/44529). When your SUDS level has gotten to a 25 or below for one scenario, create a new script with the next most difficult worst-case scenario you identified above. Be sure to follow the guidelines in "Creating an Imagery Exposure Script" to make it as effective as possible.

Scene 2: _____

_____

_____

_____

_____

_____

_____

_____

_____

_____

_____

_____

Scene 3: _____

_____

_____

_____

_____

_____

_____

_____

_____

_____

_____

_____

_____

Section Review: Key Points

- Worry itself is a type of avoidance behavior. It involves using words and language rather than facing a feared image of your worst-case scenarios coming true.

- By repeatedly facing your fears, your anxiety will decrease. Facing your fears allows you to learn that what you are so afraid of is tolerable and is unlikely to happen.

- Imagery exposure involves imagining a worst-case scenario coming true in vivid detail. It works to reduce your worry in the long term because, unlike worry, it involves confronting your fears. By staying with a feared image long enough, it will lose its power and related worries will decrease.

- When doing imagery exposure, it's important to let go of avoidance behaviors, such as distraction, changing the scene, or focusing only on the easier parts of the image.

Home Practice

- **Visualization Skills:** If you are having trouble, practice your visualization skills with neutral scenes.

- **Imagery Exposure Practice:** Do three five-minute imagery exposure exercises each day with the script you created, and track your progress on the recording form on the next page. This may feel like a lot, but consistency is the key to success with imagery exposure, so it will be worth it. Only doing it once or twice, however, is unlikely to help. The goal is to keep doing the same image until your SUDS level becomes a 25.

- **New Imagery Exposure Scripts:** Create two new scripts with the other worst-case scenarios you imagined. When your SUDS are 25 or below in response to one script, start doing exposure with the next most difficult one. If you are having difficulty creating a vivid scene for one scenario, you can try switching to another, but make sure you've given it an honest effort.

Imagery Exposure Recording Form

Track the maximum level your SUDS reaches during the exposure, and where it is at the end of the exercise. Also, rate how vivid the imagery was (shoot for > 50). Finally, mark whether you used any avoidance behaviors like distraction or focusing on the easier parts of the scene.

Date	Scenario	Peak SUDS (0–100)	End SUDS (0–100)	Vividness (0–100)	Avoidance (Yes/No)

Changing Behaviors

Let's review the cases of Jill, Elijah, and Sofia with an emphasis on their *anxiety-driven behaviors*—the behaviors they are each engaging in driven by their anxiety. We're going to use their anxiety-driven behaviors as examples throughout this module to help you generate your own behavioral change plan!

Jill

Jill has done a great job of engaging in more progressive muscle relaxation practice and challenging negative thoughts that come up throughout her workweek. However, she still spends a lot of time on the weekends worrying about the upcoming workweek. This week she has yet another presentation in front of her boss, so she's feeling particularly "on edge." She tries using her detached awareness skills to observe the worries objectively, which helps for a short period of time, but then the worries come back. Jill wants to spend her weekend focusing on things she likes, such as getting brunch with her friends and finally finishing that novel for book group, but her anxiety keeps driving her to think about work and prepare. She spends a great deal of time just opening and closing her schedule for next week in her phone and constantly refreshing her email to see if anyone from work has emailed her. She's written copious notes in her presentation slides for the presentation she has to give in front of her boss and she continually rereads the notes, but she doesn't seem able to take it all in or remember any of the material. As a result, Jill is feeling overwhelmed and worried about the upcoming week.

Elijah

Elijah has seen some progress in his avoidance and anxiety about schoolwork, largely resulting from successfully using his "rethinking thoughts" skills about the likelihood and consequences of failing his classes. By reminding himself that a grade below an A isn't a catastrophe, and by practicing mindful breathing when he worries about school, he's been able to focus more on his work and get it done on time. He's even gotten positive feedback on some recent assignments! However, he's continued to avoid looking at his credit card and student loan statements because they make him so anxious. He gets irritable whenever his girlfriend brings up finances, and he has a hard time opening up about his anxiety to her. He's become more aware of this and realizes that he has a lot of automatic thoughts about her leaving him because of his anxiety issues. This has yet to help him kick his habit of avoidance thought. In addition, he still has some difficulty sleeping and distracts himself a lot with TV in order to avoid his anxious thoughts.

Sofia

Sofia was worried constantly about the safety and well-being of her children, particularly her elder son, who just went off to college. She's been trying to practice rethinking her thoughts about his safety, but she still calls and texts him multiple times each day. After practicing the imagery exposure, she no longer assumes the worst-case scenario if her kids don't respond to her, but she will keep checking in with them until she hears back. Sofia also feels easily overwhelmed by minor things like being on time and doing errands. She feels like she never has enough time to get things done and gets worked up if she thinks she might be late to something, even though she's always punctual. Since practicing the muscle relaxation, she's noticed that her headaches and neck pain, which previously had triggered further worry, have improved. Because of this improvement, she spends less time researching possible physical ailments on the Internet, and she schedules fewer doctors' appointments for reassurance, but occasionally she will still find herself engaging in those behaviors.

The Behavioral Component of Anxiety

You can see that your workbook companions have made good progress using their skills, but one thing holding them back is that they're engaging in a lot of anxiety-driven behaviors. That might be the case for you as well. In this module, we'll focus on those anxious behaviors that tend to maintain anxiety.

As we discussed in Module 1, the behavioral part of anxiety refers to what you *do* as a result of your anxious feelings. Behaviors are typically thought of as involving an action that you can observe, such as Jill refreshing her email and checking her schedule over and over again instead of reading the book for book group or going out with her friends. However, behavior can also involve almost imperceptible or internal action. For example, Jill might also be sitting in front of her computer just thinking about what will happen if she does a bad job on the presentation next week. Jill's worry *is* the behavior in this case. We can think of worry as a behavior when it describes what you are doing in response to a situation. Rather than problem solving, which would involve trying out a strategy to make progress on her presentation, Jill is worrying. The content of her thoughts during worrying ("I'm going to do a terrible job on this presentation") make up the cognitive component of anxiety, but the *act* of worrying is a *behavior*. It's important to classify worry as well as other unhelpful behaviors as you try to change these behaviors to be more in line with your personal values and goals.

Below is the list of common behaviors associated with anxiety that we first discussed in Module 1. Again, review this list and check off any that you engage in, and add others to the list if you think of them.

☐ Procrastinating

☐ Seeking reassurance

☐ Venting

☐ Over-preparing or over-researching

☐ Worrying

☐ Checking something over and over

☐ Being extremely cautious

☐ Distracting yourself (with TV, conversation, Internet)

☐ Leaving a situation

☐ Drinking alcohol or using other drugs

☐ Keeping safety items (other people, medications) with you

☐ Refusing to delegate tasks to others

☐ Other: _____

☐ Other:_____

☐ Other: _____

Intolerance of Uncertainty

Why do we engage in these behaviors? A major reason for any anxiety-driven behavior is an intolerance of uncertainty, or the inability to deal with life's uncertainties. Let's face it: life is unpredictable. We'd love to have a crystal ball, but we don't. We want to be certain about the outcome of an event, but we can't. Intolerance of uncertainty results from the belief that uncertainty or ambiguity is a bad thing. Uncertainty by its definition is neither good nor bad, just unknown. However, it's that unknown that individuals with high anxiety perceive as being negative or threatening. Intolerance of uncertainty is the fuel for the engine of worry. Anxious people, particularly people who worry excessively, are more likely to be very intolerant of uncertainty. Just like Jill, they often try to plan and prepare for everything as a way of avoiding or eliminating uncertainty. People with generalized anxiety disorder have a greater intolerance of uncertainty than the general public or even people with other anxiety disorders. People who have high levels of intolerance to uncertainty believe that it's unacceptable that a negative event may occur, however small the probability of its occurrence. Uncertainty is viewed as negative, stressful, upsetting, and something that should be avoided.

If the general state of uncertainty is aversive and threatening, then worry becomes a strategy to mentally plan and prepare for any outcome and thus reduce uncertainty. Individuals with generalized anxiety disorder engage in safety-seeking behaviors designed to either reduce uncertainty or avoid it altogether. Examples include behaviors mentioned above (reassurance seeking, double-checking, excessive information seeking, procrastination, avoidance of novel situations). By engaging in these behaviors, they maintain the belief that uncertainty is an undesirable state that should be minimized as much as possible in order to function optimally in daily life.

Obviously, it's typical for most people to be a bit uncomfortable with uncertainty. We don't just draw out of a hat randomly for every action we take. We'd prefer to know which restaurant we're going to, that there will be a projector available for our presentation, and when a test is coming up. Having this knowledge feels much more palatable than being unprepared.

Intolerance of uncertainty is like an allergy, such as an allergy to peanuts. If you are allergic to uncertainty, even at very small doses (just a dusting of peanuts in the air) you may experience unpleasant side effects (anxiety), and the greater the uncertainty (eating a whole peanut), the more anxiety you may experience. Everyone with generalized anxiety tends to have this allergy, but the severity can vary from person to person. To examine your level of intolerance for uncertainty, consider the following questions.

1. *Make a list here of all the things you are 100 percent certain of:*

_____

_____

_____

_____

2. *Could you think of anything? Why is it so difficult to come up with things we're 100 percent certain of? Is it because there is very little we can be that certain of? Do we actually tolerate thousands, millions, of uncertainties every day without thinking about it?*

3. *If intolerance to uncertainty is the fuel for the engine of worry, then you can either choose to increase your certainty or increase your tolerance. Think about which strategy you've been using. Has it been beneficial in reducing your anxiety? Has it helped reduce anxiety about future situations? If being intolerant to uncertainty hasn't worked in reducing anxiety, what's the alternative?*

Dealing with uncertainty is an unavoidable part of daily life. Because we can't see the future, we can never be truly certain about what is going to happen. Increasing your tolerance to uncertainty is a better strategy than attempting to increase your certainty: it's always possible to become more tolerant, but it's not possible to become completely certain. So one of the goals of this treatment is to change your attitude toward uncertainty. Because worrying prevents you from discovering whether your fears actually come true, you'll be encouraged to engage in behavioral experiments that expose you to uncertainty so you can test your negative beliefs. This is accomplished by asking yourself to act "as if" you were tolerant of uncertainty. After the experiment, you'll consider whether the feared outcome came true and how you coped with it. We'll discuss this in more detail after we review avoidance as a behavior and its insidious relationship with anxiety.

Avoidance as a Behavior

Anxious behaviors are almost always failed attempts to reduce anxiety. Feeling anxious is unpleasant, so naturally we want to avoid it. We dislike uncertainty, so naturally we try to gain certainty about situations. Unfortunately, attempts to avoid anxiety or gain complete certainty are often ineffective, especially in the long term. In fact, avoidance is actually one of the primary reasons why anxiety becomes a persistent problem. To remind you how this works, let's first review our definition from Module 1 of what we mean by avoidance:

Avoidance is anything you do, or don't do, to reduce your anxiety.

What forms of avoidance do we see in Jill's example above? Check them off from the list and add any others:

☐ Procrastinating

☐ Seeking reassurance

☐ Venting

☐ Over-preparing or over-researching

☐ Worrying

☐ Checking something over and over

☐ Being extremely cautious

☐ Distracting yourself (with TV, conversation, Internet)

☐ Leaving a situation

☐ Drinking alcohol or using other drugs

☐ Keeping safety items (other people, medications) with you

☐ Refusing to delegate tasks to others

☐ Other: _____

☐ Other: _____

☐ Other: _____

☐ Other: _____

Facing Anxiety Through Behavioral Change and Exposure

Let's return now to our three components of anxiety and summarize how they influence each other. We discussed back in Module 1 how the cognitive, physical, and behavioral components of anxiety interact to form a vicious cycle of anxiety. We can see this in the figure below, which describes Jill's situation:

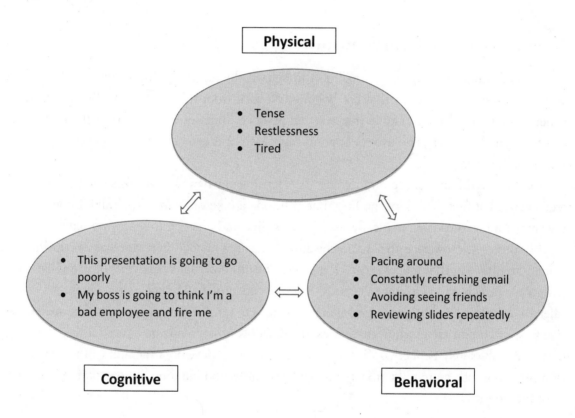

Figure 6.1. *Three Components of Anxiety (Jill)*

As we discussed in Module 5, exposure provides an opportunity for you to learn that real catastrophes are not likely to occur, even if you don't engage in avoidance or checking behaviors (for example, Jill's boss will likely not fire her even if she doesn't check her email ten times each hour). Exposure exercises give you the opportunity to practice the anxiety-management skills you've learned up to this point in everyday situations that are relevant to your anxiety. Anxious concerns are often not entirely realistic, and spending time avoiding them through worry or other means is harmful and keeping you from living your full life. It can be difficult to realize the ways that anxiety is holding you back. In Module 5, you visualized your feared scenarios and watched your anxiety decrease with repeated imagery exposure. Now you'll practice behavioral exposure; that is, you'll repeatedly choose to stop avoiding and thus test whether your feared scenarios actually come true. This will be difficult, but if you stick with it you'll see your anxiety decrease over time. Behavioral exposure is a step toward tolerating uncertainty rather than being intolerant of uncertainty.

Practicing Behavioral Exposure

To practice behavioral exposure, you'll go through all the anxiety-driven avoidance behaviors you are engaging in currently that are holding you back from fully living your life and instead generate more helpful alternatives that you can practice. Initially, it will be very challenging to resist avoidance behaviors in favor of opposite, approach-oriented behaviors; however, with practice, it becomes easier.

Exposure is difficult but rewarding. Just like learning any new skill, it takes practice and may feel awkward at first. Think of the first time you rode a bike or drove a car…did it come completely naturally to you automatically? No! It takes time and practice to reach your goals.

Be sure to acknowledge that some checking behaviors may be important or worthwhile (if you are in poor health it makes sense to engage in health-conscious behaviors or if you live in a dangerous neighborhood it makes sense to be more concerned and check more carefully on the safety of your family). The primary goal of exposure is to target fears and worries that are excessive to your current circumstances. (For example, will your job really be at stake if you don't do everything absolutely perfectly?) To target these fears, we'll develop a hierarchy of feared situations, starting with more mild anxiety-inducing scenarios and building up to situations that get at your core fear.

Creating an Anxious Behavior Hierarchy

To start challenging your anxiety, make a list of all your worry-driven behaviors. What does worrying lead you to do? What does worrying make you avoid? If you are having difficulty generating a list, look back at your past home practice assignments and pull some items from your behavior component circles. Refer to the list you generated earlier in this module; which behaviors did you check? List all these behaviors below in the first column under "Anxiety-Driven Behaviors." (A worksheet is available at http://www.newharbinger.com/44529.)

Anxiety-Driven Behaviors	Non-Anxious Behaviors	SUDS (0–100)

Next, from this list create a set of non-anxious goals (under the "Non-Anxious Behaviors" column) that are designed to replace the anxious behaviors. These non-anxious behaviors can be the opposite of avoidance; they help you approach your worries and fears head-on. Ask yourself, "If I wasn't feeling anxious about this situation, instead of the anxiety-driven behavior, what would I do?" For example, if Jill were to say to herself, "If I wasn't feeling anxious about this presentation next week, instead of staying home checking my email and rereading my slides, what would I do?" Jill's answer would be something like "Join my friends for brunch" or "Read my book group book I've been wanting to catch up on." Next, under the SUDS column, list your rating of distress (0–100) that you believe you'd feel if you were to engage in the non-anxious behavior rather than the anxiety-driven behavior in that moment. Let's take a look at Jill's completed list:

Anxiety-Driven Behaviors	Non-Anxious Behaviors	SUDS (0–100)
Procrastinating	Start within 5 minutes	60
Over-preparing	Limit preparation to 1 hour	70
Checking email repeatedly	Only check email 1x per hour	80
Pacing	Sit still	50
Worrying	Be in the present moment	70

Did you have any difficulties generating your lists? Think through what Elijah or Sofia would add to their lists and see whether any of their behaviors are the same as yours. Look back at your home practice assignments and pay particular attention to what you put in the "Behaviors" column, and see if that gives you more ideas about what to put down. Also note that this list is a work in progress, and you should pay special attention to your anxious behaviors going forward so you can keep adding to it.

Behavior Change Planning

Now that you have your hierarchy or list of non-anxious behaviors, pick about two to practice over the next week. Think ahead of time what sort of practical issues might be associated with that behavioral change item. For example, depending on what goals you set, the behavioral change may require some advance planning, such as setting up social arrangements (for example, Jill planning a brunch) or letting significant others know you are not going to be making daily calls to check in on their safety as you usually do. There are some other logistical challenges to think about; for example, some tasks can be practiced repeatedly very quickly (such as limiting texts to check on loved ones to once per day). Other tasks will have to be spread out over longer periods of time (such as once a week or allowing for social opportunities). In those instances (when the behaviors are less frequent), you might want to tackle several behavioral changes at once. Consider what anxious thoughts might come to mind as a result of the behavioral change and think about how to challenge those ahead of time. Practice each behavioral change exercise as many times as necessary for the associated anxiety to decrease at least in half or to a mild level (about 30 or less on the SUDS).

One of the main recommendations for behavioral change and exposures is being consistent! For example, let's say that Jill realizes that she will have five presentations coming up in the next month. However, she combats over-preparation for only one of the presentations by limiting her preparation time to an hour. Each of the other four times she still engages in her avoidance behavior of over-preparing. How helpful do you think that will be for Jill's anxiety? To really target her anxiety, Jill will have to be consistent in applying non-anxious behaviors that are the opposite of her avoidance strategies. It's certainly hard to do, and we need to be forgiving to ourselves if we occasionally slip up, but that's the ultimate goal. Now, let's have you try this!

Implementing Your Behavioral Change Plan

First start with smaller (lower on the hierarchy, a SUDS rating of 40 or less) behavioral change goals and build success from the momentum of accomplishing the smaller goals. Be prepared to feel anxious when you first change your behavior, but stay the course. Then afterward, review how it went. Did your anxiety eventually decrease? Did the bad outcomes you were worried about end up coming true? If something bad did happen, was it really as bad as you feared? This is the same concept as what you did in Module 4, Section II, when you reviewed the consequences of reducing worry. If you find yourself holding on to "what if" thoughts or wishing you had engaged in your anxious behavior, use your rethinking thoughts skills to further examine the validity of those thoughts. Paying attention to the way in which outcomes weren't as bad as you feared can encourage you to engage in more non-anxious behaviors. Use the Behavioral Exposure Monitoring Form at the end of this module (and at http://www.newharbinger.com/44529) to record your progress.

Section Review: Key Points

- The behavioral part of anxiety refers to what you *do* as a result of your anxious feelings.

- These behaviors are often driven by an intolerance of uncertainty. Because it's impossible to eliminate all uncertainty from our lives, we must instead learn to bolster our tolerance of uncertainty.

- Creating a hierarchy of anxiety-driven behaviors and their non-anxious behavioral counterparts helps you challenge anxiety through exposure. With continued practice, non-anxious behaviors will get easier to do and anxiety will ultimately decrease.

Home Practice

- **Continue Building Your Hierarchy:** Monitor your anxious behaviors during the week, and add any new ones you notice to your hierarchy. Then identify the corresponding non-anxious alternative behavior.

- **Behavioral Exposures:** Conduct at least three exposure exercises in this next week (using non-anxious behaviors from your hierarchy), and record how they went on the Behavioral Exposure Monitoring Form. Begin with non-anxious behaviors that have distress ratings corresponding to approximately 40 to 60 on the 0–100 scale. Stick with each exposure until your anxiety has reduced by at least 50 percent, and then afterward review whether your feared outcomes came true. Keep trying different exposures (moving up your hierarchy) and be sure to reward yourself after you avoid avoidance (and use approaching behaviors instead)!

Behavioral Exposure Monitoring Form

Date	Situation	Non-Anxious Behavior	Outcome of Behavior (Did feared consequences come true? Was it as bad as you feared?)	Peak SUDS (0–100)	End SUDS (0–100)

MODULE 7

Progress on Goals and Relapse Prevention

At the beginning of this book, we congratulated you for opening up this workbook and taking the first step toward doing something about your anxiety. Now that you've made it to the seventh and final module, even bigger congratulations are in order. We've challenged you to do some pretty difficult things: become more conscious of the way your anxious mind works, change the way you respond to your thoughts and feelings, develop new patterns of behavior, and ultimately try to establish a different relationship with anxiety. This has involved a lot of work! By sticking with it and making it this far, you've given yourself a chance to make some really meaningful changes, so give yourself a pat on the back.

Rather than teaching you a new skill or concept, in this module we're going to review the progress you've made and the skills you've learned. We'll also talk about how you can maintain your gains, and even continue to reduce the way in which anxiety interferes with your life.

Reviewing the Skills

We've introduced a lot of different strategies for responding to anxiety effectively. We've also introduced some important insights into the nature of anxiety that we hope you've taken to heart. So, let's start with a brief review of the main points and tools we've covered. If you need a refresher on any of these, we've included the module where they are covered, and encourage you to look back at those pages to remind yourself of the details.

Key Points

- **Worry vs. Problem Solving:** Worry is an unhelpful *thinking* response to a potential problem that makes your anxiety worse, even though sometimes it *feels* helpful. Problem solving is the adaptive alternative to worry and involves taking active steps toward a solution. (Module 1)

- **Avoidance Behavior:** Anxiety causes us to engage in avoidance behavior, which is anything you *do* or *don't do* to reduce anxiety. Avoidance provides short-term relief, but in the long term prevents you from learning more adaptive ways to respond to stress. (Modules 1 and 6)

- **Physical Relaxation:** Anxiety is physical as well as mental in nature. One way to reduce anxiety is to reduce the amount of physical tension in your body. (Module 2)

- **Thoughts as Hypotheses:** We form patterns in the way we automatically think about the world, and these thoughts often drive anxiety. If we slow our thinking down, treat our thoughts as hypotheses, and evaluate how realistic or useful they are, we can develop less anxiety-inducing ways of viewing situations. (Module 3)

- **Attention and Worry:** Our anxiety is impacted by where we focus our attention. By shifting our attention away from worries and toward the present moment, and by viewing our thoughts as "just thoughts," we can stop the worry cycle. (Module 4).

- **Facing Our Fears:** Repeatedly engaging in non-anxious behaviors and facing our fears helps us increase our tolerance of uncertainty and realize that the disastrous consequences we expect are unlikely to occur. (Modules 5 and 6)

Skills Covered

Skill	How to the Use Skill	Module Covered
Progressive Muscle Relaxation	Tense and relax different muscles groups in order to attain physical relaxation.	2
Mindful Breathing	Inhale (5 seconds), hold breath (3 seconds), and exhale (5 seconds) while focusing on the breath.	2
Challenging Probability Overestimation	Evaluate the evidence for and against an anxious thought, assessing the actual probability of the feared outcome occurring, and identifying a more realistic alternative thought.	3
Challenging Catastrophic Thinking	Determine the actual severity of a feared outcome, identify how you'd cope if the outcome came true, and generate a more realistic interpretation of the situation.	3
Detached Awareness	Observe your anxious thoughts as just thoughts without assigning particular importance to them. You can do this using visual imagery (a train passing through a station, leaves on a stream, thoughts written on sand).	4
Worry Postponement	Postpone all worries to a specified 20- to 30-minute period of the day where you allow yourself to worry.	4
Imagery Exposure	Repeatedly imagine worst-case scenarios using visual imagery for 5-minute intervals until the anxiety becomes minimal.	5
Behavioral Exposure	Engage in non-anxious behaviors (approach feared situations rather than avoid) in order to learn that anxiety-driven behaviors are not necessary to prevent feared outcomes.	6

Reviewing Your Progress

Progress often comes gradually, so sometimes we don't realize just how much we've changed. To help with this, think back to how your anxiety impacted your life when you first opened this workbook. Take a look at your home practice worksheets in Module 1, including the two self-monitoring forms, and the list of areas of interference and distress caused by anxiety. Is anxiety interfering with your life in the same way? How were you handling your anxiety then compared to now? Do the same thoughts and situations trigger anxiety as before, or do you notice you have different ways of responding to anxiety now?

You should also take a look at the goals you made for yourself in Module 1, along with what it would look like if you met those goals. Check off anything from your goals worksheet that you've been able to accomplish. Then sum up your progress in the space below by writing down the areas that you've seen the most improvement in.

In addition, it's important to pay attention to what helped you improve, as that's going to be something you'll want to keep up. For example, if you are no longer as stressed at work, is this because you are doing PMR each morning? Because you can challenge beliefs about the catastrophic consequences of negative feedback from your boss? Or because you've done behavioral exposures surrounding perfectionism and reassurance seeking? Or perhaps some combination of these? Write down the skills or insights that you see as the main driving forces behind your major improvements, as these will form an important part of your relapse prevention plan.

Areas of Greatest Improvement	What Contributed to This Improvement
1.	
2.	
3.	

Maintaining Your Gains

When people see reductions in their anxiety levels, it's natural to wonder whether those gains will last. The good news is that typically people do maintain improvement after a course of treatment. This is because it's hard to unlearn the skills and insights you've developed. In adopting the skills taught in this workbook, you've actually changed the way your brain works, and those changes don't change back easily!

Nonetheless, it can be helpful to have a plan in place for ensuring that your improvements last. An important part of this is understanding that there will be fluctuations in your anxiety, and to make sure not to catastrophize any increases in anxiety. In other words, know that there is a difference between a lapse and a relapse, and realize how you can prevent the latter:

Lapse: A *temporary* increase in symptoms because of increase in stress or not using skills

Relapse: An extended period of increased anxiety, decreased functioning, and the complete absence of skill use

Lapses are to be expected. In Module 1, we talked about stress (disruptions from the status quo) being a major contributor to problematic anxiety. There will inevitably be times of increased stress in your life, and it's possible that these could lead to a lapse, especially if you forget or are unsure of how to use your skills in response to the stress.

The most important thing to do if you notice a lapse is to figure out what strategies you can apply to better respond to your stress and anxiety. Increased stress doesn't inevitably lead to problematic anxiety if you respond to it effectively, and you now have a whole host of tools at your disposal to help you do so. So if you are experiencing an increase in symptoms, come back to Module 1 to remind yourself of your options.

It's also important to watch out for any thoughts that you are completely slipping when you experience a lapse, as this sort of catastrophizing can start a worry cycle that will increase anxiety even further. If you find yourself worrying about relapse, look back at the definition. Relapses happen because of a *complete* absence of skill use. Whether you use your skills or not is totally in your control, and you won't relapse if you keep using what you've learned.

Identifying High-Risk Lapse Areas

You can also decrease the likelihood of both lapses and relapses by planning ahead. Think about your life in the next six months to a year, and identify any situations or potential stressors that might put you at high risk of lapsing. Thinking back to your workbook companions: this might be the exam period at the end of the semester for Elijah, or managing a romantic relationship for Jill. A high-risk situation can also be something that's not planned or expected, but has caused severe levels of anxiety in the past. For example, Sofia knows that when she catches even a minor cold, this triggers intense anxiety about having more serious medical issues.

Once you've identified your high-risk situations, think about the anxiety-driven behaviors you might engage in that could make things worse, as these are the things you'll want to watch out for. Then you can identify the skillful, effective behaviors you could use to apply in such a situation instead. See below for an example with Sofia.

High-Risk Situations	Anxiety-Driven Behaviors to Watch Out For	Skillful Behaviors to Reduce Risk of Lapse
Getting sick; will trigger thoughts about having a serious illness	• Seeking reassurance from husband • Internet research • Repeated doctors' visits • Avoiding daily activities	• Detached awareness to remind myself that thoughts about illness are just thoughts, not reality • Imagery exposure to having terminal illness

Now fill out the boxes below with your own high-risk situations, anxiety-driven behaviors, and skillful behaviors.

High-Risk Situations	Anxiety-Driven Behaviors to Watch Out For	Skillful Behaviors to Reduce Risk of Lapse
1.		
2.		
3.		

Areas for Continued Improvement

As you went through the process of reviewing your progress, you likely noticed that, while you've seen improvements, there are still some things you'd like to work on. This is totally normal, and you shouldn't feel disappointed! Many people who receive therapy actually make further improvements after treatment is over as they continue applying the skills in their daily lives. The nice thing about where you are now is that you have the skills you need, so all you have to do is make a plan for how best to use them.

To make that plan, identify the most important areas of improvement for you going forward. You might draw from goals you made at the beginning of the workbook that you have yet to meet. You can also look at your imagery exposure and behavioral exposure hierarchies from the last two modules for good ideas. Once you've identified these areas of improvement, return to the list of skills and key points at the beginning of this module to help you generate ideas about how best to continue to see progress.

Areas for Continued Improvement	How I Can Achieve This
1.	
2.	
3.	

Concluding Thoughts

Anxiety is a challenging problem to tackle because even though it can cause a lot of difficulties, it's also a normal part of life. As a result, reducing problematic anxiety doesn't mean never feeling anxious; it means getting to a place where anxiety no longer interferes with the things you care about in your life. In looking forward, we hope that you'll keep this perspective in mind, as it can help you maintain a healthy relationship with anxiety. That relationship isn't one where you avoid feeling anxious at all costs. It's one where you are able to identify when your anxiety is getting in the way of things or is causing undue distress, and then are able to use your skills in a way that helps you live your life more freely. Sometimes that will mean confronting situations that bring on anxiety in the short term, but in the long term that's where some of the most powerful changes come from. Having gone through this book, you now have the power to deal with anxiety differently, so good luck as you move forward in your life.

Module Review: Key Points

- You've done a lot of hard work and now have a lot of skills at your disposal. The key to maintaining your gains and seeing continued improvement is to keep using those skills!

- Lapses are temporary periods of increased anxiety, and are to be expected. To reduce lapses and prevent them from turning into relapses, identify situations where your anxiety is more likely to return, and plan ahead for how you can effectively cope with them.

- Transforming your anxious mind is a long-term process, and it's normal to feel like there are more gains to be made. Keep in mind that anxiety is also a normal part of life, but by using your skills you can prevent it from interfering with the things you care about.

References

Aviation Safety. 2018. "Statistical Summary of Commercial Jet Airplane Accidents Worldwide Operations: 1959–2017." *Boeing Commercial Airplanes*. www.boeing.com/news/techissues/pdf /statsum.pdf

Beck, A. T. 1976. *Cognitive Therapy and the Emotional Disorders*. New York: International Universities Press.

Carpenter, J. K., L. A. Andrews, S. M. Witcraft, M. B. Powers, J. A. Smits, and S. G. Hofmann. 2018. "Cognitive Behavioral Therapy for Anxiety and Related Disorders: A Meta-Analysis of Randomized Placebo-Controlled Trials." *Depression and Anxiety* 35: 502–514.

Craske, M. G., and D. H. Barlow. 2006. *Mastery of Your Anxiety and Worry: Client Workbook*. 2nd ed. New York: Oxford University Press.

Hayes, S. C. (with S. Smith). 2005. *Get Out of Your Mind and Into Your Life: The New Acceptance and Commitment Therapy*. Oakland, CA: New Harbinger.

Hofmann, S. G., A. T. Sawyer, A. A. Witt, and D. Oh. 2010. "The Effect of Mindfulness-Based Therapy on Anxiety and Depression: A Meta-Analytic Review." *Journal of Consulting and Clinical Psychology* 78: 169–183.

Locke, E. A., and G. P. Latham. 2002. "Building a Practically Useful Theory of Goal Setting and Task Motivation: A 35-Year Odyssey." *American Psychologist* 57: 705–717.

Webb, T. L., and P. Sheeran. 2006. "Does Changing Behavioral Intentions Engender Behavior Change? A Meta-Analysis of the Experimental Evidence." *Psychological Bulletin* 132: 249–268.

Wells, A., and S. Cartwright-Hatton. 2004. "A Short Form of the Metacognitions Questionnaire: Properties of the MCQ-30." *Behaviour Research and Therapy* 42: 385–396.

Stefan G. Hofmann, PhD, is a professor in Boston University's department of psychological and brain sciences clinical program, where he directs the Psychotherapy and Emotion Research Laboratory (PERL). His research focuses on the mechanism of treatment change—translating discoveries from neuroscience into clinical applications, emotions, and cultural expressions of psychopathology. He is past president of the Association for Behavioral and Cognitive Therapies (ABCT), and the International Association for Cognitive Psychotherapy (IACP). He is also editor in chief of *Cognitive Therapy and Research*, and associate editor of *Clinical Psychological Science*. He has authored numerous books, including *An Introduction to Modern CBT* and *Emotion in Therapy*.

Foreword writer **Judith S. Beck, PhD**, is director of the Beck Institute for Cognitive Behavior Therapy, clinical associate professor of psychology in psychiatry at the University of Pennsylvania, and past president of the Academy of Cognitive Therapy. Daughter of influential founder of cognitive therapy, Aaron T. Beck, Beck resides in Bala Cynwyd, PA. She is author of *The Beck Diet Solution*.

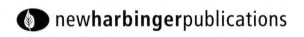